RECLAIM THE JOY
of Motherhood
How I Defeated Postpartum Depression

BY PAMELA K ZIMMER

RECLAIM THE JOY
of **Motherhood**

How I Defeated Postpartum Depression

BY PAMELA K ZIMMER

Editorial and Production Management: Christine, Ink.
Cover and Interior Design: Ali Alden, Dexter Design House
Cover Photography: Courtney Spangler
Author Photo: Alina Vincent Photography

Printed in the United States of America

ISBN-10: 0991294300
ISBN-13: 978-0-9912943-0-5

TABLE OF CONTENTS

TABLE OF CONTENTS (CONT.)

ACKNOWLEDGEMENTS

I would like to take a moment here to share with you a couple of the mentors who inspired me to follow this path. There are many amazing women out there who are speaking out about PPD, or helping guide others toward new levels of happiness and success. In my own life and transformation, I have been heavily influenced by two of them in particular.

Katherine Stone is a beautiful, strong soul who tirelessly shares information and hope for Postpartum Depression recovery, and has been doing it for over a decade as of this writing. Her work at Postpartum Progress, Inc., a nonprofit organization dedicated to maternal mental health, has been a huge influence in the lives of many women, myself included. I follow her religiously; she is an inspiration to be bold and brave. I hope that other women will see in me what I see in Katherine: a resource for information and inspiration, with the addition of specific tools and programs for recovery.

And speaking of the tools and programs, I was deeply influenced by Lisa Sasevich, whose instructional program helped me to determine exactly how to do what I wanted to do. By looking first at the value I wanted to provide for women, and then working backward, I was able to come up with programs that work smoothly and flow effortlessly, helping you get the greatest possible value from The HAPPY Mommy Method™.

In regards to writing this book, and my entire healing journey for that matter, there are several other people I want to acknowledge and thank. I want to thank Marlena Smoot, my doula, for caring about me and my family enough to push me to get the help I needed. I want to thank my doctors, Dr. Steve Thompson and Carol Lindsay, for listening to me and supporting me throughout my recovery.

I want to thank and acknowledge Kristin Hodson, Valerie McManus and Stacey Glaesmann for contributing their time and expertise on Postpartum Depression, and for allowing me to supplement my research with theirs.

I could not have written this book without the support, love and encouragement of my father, Fred, and my friends, who believed in me and who helped watch my boys for me when I needed a break, or just came to be with me as I was going through my PPD, and then later when I needed extra time and space to write this book. Special thanks and acknowledgement to Elisa and Courtney who shared their experience of my PPD and allowed me to include it in this book.

A big thank you to Ali Alden for the beautiful cover design, and Christine Whitmarsh and her amazing editorial team: Jessica, Nathan and Michelle. You all collectively held me up and kept me going, you held me accountable and reminded me of why I was doing what I was doing. You believed in me and gave me space to write when I needed to write and a safe place to be completely vulnerable and tell my story, tears and all. I know there are many more people in my life whom supported and encouraged me, but

I can't possibly list them all here. So to you, I say thank you for helping me achieve this dream.

Lastly, to my husband, Will, thank you for your unconditional support and love. Without you I would not be where I am today, literally. You are my rock, my constant and I love you with all my heart. To my two boys, Zackery and Brayden, you both brighten my day each and every morning and I am so happy and proud to be your (happy) Mommy.

PROLOGUE

Everything's Going To Be Okay

"I'm not afraid of storms, for I'm learning to sail my ship."

-Louisa May Alcott

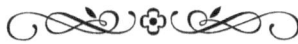

I am laughing out loud, arms outstretched toward my son as he flies through the air. He shrieks in joy, clutching the swing with his little hands, and on the neighboring swing, his brother erupts in giggles. I can't help but join in. The sunlight bounces off their fine, tousled hair, their chubby elbows, their sweet faces. The warm breeze embraces me and I want to hug it right back. I think to myself, "This is what joy feels like." And then I push the swing again, sending my beloved boy high into the sky.

It has been three years since I was diagnosed with Postpartum Depression, and one year since I stopped my medication. There was never a specific moment when I suddenly "got happy." It wasn't like a switch flipped and flooded my life with light again. It was so much more subtle and gradual, like a long summer sunrise after a sleepless night. Some days are better than others, but lately, most of them are good.

When you're depressed, it's like you're in a fog and you just can't see what is going on. Your senses are dulled. You can't keep things straight from minute to minute. You can't make decisions, because it's too hard to weigh the options. Do I want coffee, or do I want tea? Do I want ice cubes in my water glass? It might sound crazy, but a couple of years ago, I could not handle those decisions—at all. It took every little ounce of my strength to focus on the one task I had to do, and that was hard enough.

Even worse, as much as I loved my happy little boys, it was so hard to be the mom I felt like I needed to be. I was constantly worried about what I was supposed to be doing for them—so worried, that I basically paralyzed myself in indecision. I knew that my sons Zackery and Brayden were the reason I needed to get out of bed every morning, and I did it out of necessity. Whether it was breastfeeding Brayden or making sure Zack was where he needed to be, I did what I had to do, and beyond that, I really couldn't make even the simplest decision.

It's kind of terrifying when your mind doesn't work. But inside my foggy brain, I didn't realize that things were seriously wrong. If you had told me I wasn't happy, I probably would have said you just didn't understand—I'm just a person who cries a lot, and I have a lot going on. Well, now I have gained some understanding, and let me tell you: I still cry sometimes! But not over untied shoes or (dare I say it) spilled milk. No longer do I cry because I don't want to get out of bed and deal with the prospect of making decisions all day long.

Today, I got up with a smile. It was easy: I was excited to hang out with my sons, and could not wait to just spend time with them. The decision to go to the park was a simple one, because I knew we would have fun. And now, pushing them on the swings while they yell in delight, I am not worried at all. The cloud has lifted, and I remember what it is like to be me: Pamela Zimmer, a strong, intelligent woman with a beautiful family. I feel brave enough to handle anything that might happen at the park today. My chest feels clear, I am breathing deeply and my eyes are taking in all the colors of the world. I feel joy with all five of my senses!

A scraped knee and some fruit snacks later, we stroll back across the fresh-cut grass, which is dotted with dandelions and clover. Zack and Brayden are talking over each other to tell me about everything they see: birds, dog poop, motorcycles, clouds that look like ice cream... Their growing minds see every detail as new and exciting, and I try to look at the world around us in the same way.

I can see even more than they can, in fact. I see them growing and learning in every moment. I see the fading sunlight splashing, yellow and pink, on their faces. I see their eyes turn to me, full of love and trust. They are happy, too: now I know the difference. And when they laugh, I laugh right back.

When we get back to the house, Will is home from work. His eyes brighten as his sons run through the door. "Daddy!!!" they yell. He scoops his little men up in his arms, and I see the three of them in the past, present and future—my beautiful boys.

Will puts down the boys, and they head for the couch. He turns to me. "Hi hon, how was the park?"

"Great," I say. I know I am beaming, my cheeks flushed and glowing. "You know what is really cool?"

"What?"

"Being happy for no reason."

Will's face lights up with a huge grin. He grabs me and envelops me in a bear hug.

For so long, I thought that only perfection would do. I had to be Super Mom and do everything just right, or it would all fall apart. But now, here, in the arms of my husband and with my boys in the next room, I see it all so differently. It doesn't matter if the laundry is dirty or if the kitchen table is messy. It doesn't matter if I make a mistake or can't do everything on my list today. Ultimately, those things make no difference at all. Either you're happy, or you're not; laundry has no bearing on the issue. The thing holding us all together is our love, and that is the only thing we need.

My name is Pamela Zimmer, and I beat Postpartum Depression. It was a long, hard journey, but I did it. And I just have one message for you, whoever you are: Everything's going to be okay.

INTRODUCTION

My Wish For You

"The thing that is really hard, and really amazing, is giving up on being perfect and beginning the work of being yourself."

-Anna Quindlen

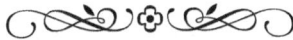

Did you know that Postpartum Depression (PPD) is the most common complication of pregnancy and childbirth? It is estimated to affect as many as one in every five new moms. And yet, I was completely certain that it would never happen to me. Maybe you feel the same way; many, many women never report their symptoms.

You might also feel like things aren't that bad—like it might just be the Baby Blues. Even when I was in the throes of PPD, I honestly didn't think I was depressed. I thought I was tired, just like every new mom. Maybe a little more tired than most, but it was something I could fix. I could do better. I even thought my exhaustion was, in some way, my own fault.

If this sounds familiar to you, then I really hope you will keep reading. This book is based on my own recovery from PPD, but it isn't really for me; it's for YOU. I want you to know that you are not alone (no matter how much it may feel like it!), that what's happening is real, and that it's not your fault. I want you to realize that it can and will get better, and that you can get help. I want to help. And I believe that I can help, because I know exactly what you are going through. I've been to the darkest of the dark places, and I'm not afraid of them any more. I can show you how to find the light again.

I would never wish upon anyone the darkness, the loneliness, or the shame I experienced while going through my Postpartum Depression, but I believe that everything happens for a reason. If I had never gone through what I did, if I had never fought with all my body and soul, if I had never healed, I would not have my story. In my mind, the reason I had to experience Postpartum Depression was so that I could become the voice for other women going through it who haven't yet found their own inner strength.

The rush of hormones a woman experiences during and after pregnancy and childbirth is powerful, but Postpartum Depression can be triggered by more than just hormones. It can occur after a combination of external, environmental factors or stressors, such as death, closing a business, bankruptcy, pregnancy, and birth.

I believe my depression started years before my diagnosis, with the death of my mother, and it grew and grew as my life changed and transformed through cumulative trauma and stress. I believe it festered inside of me like an emotional tumor, spreading like cancer until it was too much for my body to handle on its own. There was nothing I could have done to predict or prevent the onset of depression. There was no way for me to know that the hormones of pregnancy and birthing Brayden, coupled with the extreme exhaustion and fatigue of having a newborn, were just enough to tip me over the edge into darkness. Here I was, at home with one of the most precious gifts I had ever received, and I was terrified. I didn't know what to do. I didn't know anything. A war was raging in my head. At one time, I felt that I was losing the war, but in the end I won—and gained immeasurable wisdom and strength from my victory over the darkness.

Writing this book has been a big part of my own healing process. It became a mission for me: to tell my story with an open and vulnerable heart, instead of shamefully hiding it away. I got it all out there—the fear, the confusion, the grief, and the pain. Also, I documented the process of healing, of reclaiming my joy, and finally becoming myself again. I can still take myself right back to those dark places, and feel exactly where I was when things were at their worst. But now, after writing my story, I can snap myself right back out of it and into my happy life again.

I haven't read every book on PPD, but the ones I have read are all so sad, or dry and clinical—they almost made me feel worse. That's not the true story of PPD! The reality is that it doesn't last forever. You WILL get better, and there IS help out there for you. Knowing what I know now, I endeavor to bring awareness of Postpartum Depression and change the perception that it is bad, shameful and hopeless. Why should it be? It happens naturally to a huge number of women. It is not uncommon and it is definitely not your fault.

I have resolved to keep an open heart and to always be honest and vulnerable with you, because I believe that the most important thing I can accomplish with my life—other than being a loving mother and wife to my beautiful family—is to raise awareness of PPD, and help women like you find their way back to joy and happiness. I wrote this book because it's the one I wanted to read when I was hurting, and because I want you to feel the possibilities of joy and happiness, just around the corner.

In this book, I will clarify for you the difference between the Baby Blues and Postpartum Depression. I will help you understand the seriousness of this illness, and the reality that it can be treated and does get better. I will candidly share my journey with you so you can see how the elements of depression can unfold and build over time, how the voices in our heads can create doubt, fear, guilt, insecurity, and inner turmoil. But most importantly, I will show you how I defeated Postpartum Depression and equip you with the steps and tools to help you beat it, too!

I am not a medical professional or a trained expert on pregnancy and childbirth. In fact, I am deeply grateful for the support I received from my doula and my doctor, and throughout this book I will urge you to find qualified sources of treatment. It is important to note that, while I commonly refer to "your doctor," I understand and accept your ability to choose a course of health and wellness care that works for you. That may involve traditional Western medicine, or it may be any other approach of your choosing. When I talk about doctors, remember that I am simply referring to the expert(s) guiding your physical and mental treatment.

I have asked three additional experts to contribute their insights and research to this book. They are Kristin Hodson, founder of The Healing Group; Valerie McManus, a social worker and psychotherapist; and Stacey Glaesmann, a wellness consultant. All three women have extensive backgrounds working with women experiencing postpartum challenges, and I believe you will find their insights deeply helpful.

I also know from experience that, in order to truly reclaim the joy of motherhood, you have to heal yourself on every level. That is what I believe is missing from all the other books I've read on PPD: the difficult and deeply rewarding process of figuring out who you are, and becoming that person.

What makes you happy? Would you like to find out, and feel joy again? I want that for you, from the bottom of my heart. If you are ready, here is how you can get the most out of this book:

Don't give up hope. You are not going through this alone any more! Read the whole book, without skimming over or skipping any parts. It's a complete story of healing and self-discovery, and every piece will help you in a different way. Stick with it and trust me that I will guide you through the process to reclaim your own hope and happiness. Even if you are feeling totally hopeless and afraid, or angry and worn out—I understand, and I've been there. I will help you find the courage to get help. Let me take you on this journey as your friend, your companion, and your mentor. And if you ever feel like you need to talk to me beyond what's in this book, I hope you will reach out. I promise to be there for you however I can.

My wish for you—whoever you are, out there reading this—is that you will identify with my story and find new hope for your future. It will get better, and you will become so much more in touch with the important things in life, the things that bring you joy.

Are you ready to reclaim the joy of motherhood? Let's begin our journey.

SECTION I

What Is Happening To Me?

CHAPTER ONE

Whispers Take Root

*"The greater your capacity to love, the greater
your capacity to feel the pain."*

- Jennifer Aniston

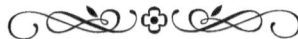

When my husband Will and I first began to talk of starting a family, I knew that getting pregnant would either happen right away for me, or it would take a long time. I wasn't a doctor, and I had no logical reasoning other than my gut feeling—but nonetheless, I believed it would either be quick, or I would be in for a long haul.

My mother once told me that I am a very determined person: whatever I put my mind to, I make it happen. It's absolutely true: I've been deeply driven since the day I was born. But I am also deeply and sometimes uncontrollably emotional. When something affects me, it affects me for a long time. Maybe that's why I was so sure that, if I couldn't get pregnant right away, it would be a long and difficult process—because that's just how things have always gone for me.

Reclaim the Joy of Motherhood

I have many happy memories of my childhood in Foster City, California, but I also remember that my parents were very strict. My father worked long hours and traveled a lot for his job as an international service manager at Apple; sometimes he would come home and continue working late into the evening. He expected the same dedication from his two daughters, and was constantly grilling us about our homework and our grades. Mom was right there with him—they were a good team—but she was also the emotional center of our family: a loving person who was always there to make things better when we were hurt or worried. My sister Susan and I always felt loved, happy, and taken care of, but we were not an openly affectionate family. Our parents respected us and our abilities, and they believed we could do anything we wanted in life; their support more often took the form of encouragement instead of affection. The most important thing, above all else, was to do your best. And you could always, always do just a little better.

My parents gave us much less freedom in our day-to-day lives than other kids had, but they also provided us with endless enriching experiences. We traveled the world and even lived in France for two years when I was in middle school. We learned so much about the important things in life—and we were also dedicated students. I always got straight A's and didn't really need to study. But I was painfully shy. I longed to be popular and well-liked, and usually wasn't.

I remember, when we came back from our two years abroad, that we moved back into our old house and the girl who had been my best friend lived on the same street. For weeks I stared out the window at her while she played outside, scared to talk to her in case she had forgotten who I was. When I finally worked up the courage, she laughed at me. "I saw you watching from your window," she said. "Why didn't you come say hi?"

That was my freshman year of high school, and it started out pretty rocky. I was overwhelmed with anxiety, loneliness, and sadness. My emotions were so strong, but I didn't feel like I could share them with anyone. I started acting out: an attempt to run away (thankfully thwarted when my mom caught me throwing a suitcase out the window); cutting myself; and even some thoughts of suicide. I really just wanted to have friends, but I couldn't control people's feelings toward me in the way I could control my grades. Over time, though, things started to turn around. I got involved in sports at school, and started to feel like I had a role to play in the fragile drama of high school social life. I made new friends on the team and in my classes. People did like me after all, and school got a lot more fun.

By the time I graduated high school I was doing really well. I had made some close friendships (which I still have to this day!) at a new school, where I was excelling in math. My grades were still high, and I could have my pick of colleges. I knew what I wanted to do: the perfect combination of emotion and logic, art and math. I wanted to be an architect.

And that's just what I did. I was an excellent student who would really beat myself up for getting anything less than an A. I was one of the few women in my architecture program, which gave me some extra clout with the male students. I joined a sorority, and by my final year of college had risen to become its president. It wasn't easy, but I finally had everything: the grades and the friendship. School was what defined me in a lot of ways, and when I graduated I needed to keep that structure and ambition in my life. I went straight out and got a job as a drafter, putting in endless hours for a local architecture office.

By the age of thirty, I really had it all. I had become the youngest woman in the area to get my architect's license, passing all ten exams in an unheard of fourteen months. I had co-founded my own architecture firm. I owned my house and my car, too. I was self-sufficient, independent, and totally able to take care of myself. I could do whatever I wanted! Just one problem: I was about four years behind on my life plan. By now, according to my calculations, I should have been married with kids. Again, just like in high school, there was something I didn't have control over and, despite all my successes, I was starting to feel like I was failing.

When I first met Will on a blind date, I didn't think he was the one for me. I was hung up on the wrong guy, and besides, I was a strong and independent woman who didn't really need a nice guy like Will. But we kept running into each other, and a few months later we hung out one-on-one again.

There was one thing I had always told my friends about what I was looking for in a partner. "I want him to be able to go camping and ride motorcycles one day, and then go to the opera the next,"

I would tell them. On my first date with Will, we had gone dirt bike riding. Now, over a casual spaghetti dinner, he asked me what I was doing that Friday.

"Why?" I asked.

"Because I have tickets to the opera, want to go?"

It didn't take long after that for me to understand that I had actually found the perfect guy. I knew he was the one. The next year was a whirlwind: we fell head over heels for each other, and just as we were planning a bright future, tragedy struck.

My mom, who had been struggling with lupus for several years, suddenly got severely ill and wound up in the hospital. Her diagnosis was a horrible shock: not just lupus, but leukemia as well. It was incurable. My mother would not survive this illness.

My emotions were going in every direction: I was so happy, so sad, so worried. Meanwhile, my biological clock was sounding five alarms, ringing and bouncing with flashing lights and sirens. I knew I was ready to get married and have kids, and I wanted to do it right away. I was racing against time, and time was winning. When Will proposed, we set a date for just three months later, and were married in November of 2005. I was thirty-one years old.

A few months later, we started trying for our first baby. I didn't know much about getting pregnant, but I knew about my monthly cycle, and that we needed to have sex only when I was ovulating— fourteen days after menstruation begins. So we had our first "try" and surprise! My next period didn't show up on time.

Reclaim the Joy of Motherhood

Could it have truly happened this first time? Were we really pregnant? Was a baby actually already growing inside me? I decided it was. I was nervous and excited, like a little girl on her birthday about to open piles of presents beautifully wrapped in silver and white paper with the most delicately tied bows of sparkling pink shear ribbon. This little girl didn't know what was inside those presents, but she knew they were gifts just for her. What a wonderful feeling!

I started spotting two days later. I wasn't pregnant, just late. I shed a few tears of disappointment and resolved to get pregnant next month—as if I was in control of it, and could simply add "get pregnant" to my shopping list and pick it up at the grocery store on my way home from work.

May and June came and went with the same precise routine, and already the process was losing its romance. It wasn't dreamy or enchanting like in movies or romance novels. Conception had been reduced to a task-oriented, calculated schedule with no spontaneity or excitement other than the anticipated result of making a baby. I desperately wanted babies. I was determined to have a tiny little soul growing inside my belly. I longed to be pregnant. I yearned to experience that miracle.

For Independence Day, Will and I drove down to visit my parents in Foster City. I remember sitting on the bed in the guest room of my parent's house when my mom walked in.

"What's wrong?" she asked.

Through the tears in my eyes, I replied, "I just got my period."
I told her that I was starting to feel like it would never happen.
I deserved to be pregnant; I needed it. But the stars just weren't
aligned.

"It will happen in time," she consoled me. Her love was so strong,
even through the sickness that made her body weaker all the time.
I knew we did not have all the time in the world, but I wanted to
believe her. I was distraught with worry.

The next day, we all went out to my hometown's traditional
Independence Day celebration. We had a marvelous time at the
fireman's pancake breakfast, playing carnival games, strolling
through the arts and craft booths, and listening to music from the
bandstand. There wasn't anything more cheery, happy, or fun than
to spend a beautiful, sunshiny day celebrating the Fourth of July
with my family. But as fireworks bloomed in the sky, there was still
one question weighing on my mind: Will I ever get pregnant?

Some couples have to endure months, even years, of hormone
therapy, injections, and medical procedures—and sometimes it's
all for nothing. My mother suffered two debilitating miscarriages
before my parents decided to adopt my sister Susan; it wasn't
until a few months after they brought Susan home that mom got
pregnant with a happy accident: me. I am so grateful that Will and
I never knew the pain that so many other couples go through. Still,
month after month, I could not conceive and I was starting to get
really scientific (and superstitious) about it. I tried propping my
bottom up on a pillow after sex, avoiding going to the bathroom,

only having sex in missionary position…and then a friend introduced me to Taking Charge of Your Fertility by Toni Weschler.

The book was thick. Packed full of information and various charts, complete with an accompanying CD of software I could download onto my computer. Within several days, I had read that book cover to cover. The amount of knowledge I gained was unreal. There's a saying, "You don't know what you don't know." Without going into details, I didn't know a lot! I used the software and began charting everything from my basal body temperature to the consistency of my vaginal fluid and the location of my cervix. I had never even been aware of these factors, let alone how vital a role they would play in Will and I finally conceiving. Slowly, I started to regain confidence and restore my faith that I might actually be able to get pregnant.

Now it was November, and I was sure that this was going to be the month. I believed that charting was the key. I was determined; I would be getting pregnant soon. But, to my dismay, November ended up just like all the other months: a big disappointment. The elated feeling of the little girl on her birthday was far gone—a long-forgotten, buried memory replaced with a little girl being punished and told to sit in a dark, cold, lonely room for all of eternity. Just like I'd done so many years ago as a child, I sat in my shame and looked out the window at the bright future I had dreamed. It was so close, I could almost touch it—but just like when I was a child watching my best friend play outside, I felt like that happiness didn't belong to me. Maybe I didn't deserve it at all. Little did I know the seeds I was planting in my mind.

Then December came, and my mother took a turn for the worse. She was in the hospital again, and this time it was much more serious. She was dying.

I recall driving down the road one wintry day, my mind in a heavy, melancholy fog. I don't remember where I was going, or even really how I got there. All I remember is this unwelcome thought flashing into my mind. It wasn't a memory, it wasn't something I suddenly needed to do. It was a question. It was the most frightening, taunting, lingering question I had ever been asked. Even worse, the question seemed to come from my own soul. "Would you trade your mother's life to be pregnant?" it whispered, like a crafty snake wanting to cut me an eternal deal. I could never answer the question, let alone ponder it. But it haunted me. I would never even pose such a question…where did this voice come from?

My father, sister, Will, and I were all there at my mother's side when she peacefully passed away and journeyed up to Heaven. I had written her one last, loving note, and I kept it now. Later as we went through her things, I found her old, vintage eyeglass case, with yellow and gold beads sewn all over the faded turquoise fabric that had protected her cats-eye glasses. I tucked the note inside the case, and took them both with me. To this day, I sleep with them inside my pillowcase every night, a connection to my mother that I will never lose.

My mother's death was the most devastating experience I had ever endured. According to her wish, we waited until after the holidays

to hold her memorial service. Planning the memorial gave me a
way to stay busy, but on the day of the event, I lost control. Amid
the outpouring of love and support from family and friends, I
could not stop crying. Though I was surrounded by people who
cared, I felt so alone and lost. Forget about getting pregnant. My
mother was gone!

After this, Will started noticing changes in me. I became more
distant and withdrawn. After having lost control over my emotions
at the memorial service, I wrenched down an emotional iron
curtain. I was still grieving deeply inside, but I felt like I needed to
put up a strong front—for my family, and for myself. I was facing
a new reality without my mom for support. In true Pamela form, I
held my feelings in and moved on.

The week after the service we were back at home in Truckee,
California, and I was packing for a prescheduled week-long
trip where I would be staffing and serving as a volunteer for a
leadership and personal development organization. I made a
mental note of being late with my period, but chalked it up to the
emotional stress of just having lost my mother.

My medicine cabinet was equipped with a plethora of neatly stored
home pregnancy tests, and Will suggested I take one. I didn't really
want to, fearing I would be disappointed yet again. But I talked
myself into it. I needed to know whether or not to pack tampons
for my trip! I decided to wait until the end of the day, before going
to bed; that way, if it was negative like it had been so many times
before, I wouldn't endure an entire day of saddening failure.

Will and I had finished cleaning up from dinner, and he was

getting ready to take our dog, Aussie, out for an evening walk. He ushered me into the bathroom and directed me to take the test. I heard the pitter-patter of four little paws running down the front steps in excitement as the bathroom door closed. Well, here we go again. I sat down on the toilet to pee on a stick.

The directions say to wait several minutes before looking at the stick to determine the results. I had certainly spent my fair share of time—cumulatively what seemed like hours—waiting for that second pink line to appear to confirm a positive pregnancy test. I had stared at the little window so many times, willing with all my might for a positive line to just manifest itself. I had willed myself into believing that even the faintest, tiniest, almost invisible little line my eyes could claim to see would be the line that announced the sign of life within me. Every time, I would get my hopes up so high, only to be crushed back down by a suffocating weight when I realized that I was still not pregnant.

This time it was different. Before I was even able to begin the countdown, the second line appeared. This was quicker than I could have imagined. It was dark, bold, and clearer than the line next to it. I couldn't believe it. Was this really happening? Was it true? Were my eyes playing tricks on me like they had done so many times before? I was breathless. I was speechless. Oh, my God! I was pregnant!

I ran to the front door, opened it, and stood at the top of the steps waiting for Will to come back from his walk with Aussie. I could hardly contain my excitement. It took every bit of energy and willpower I had not to fly down the steps and go running up the street to meet them. After what seemed like an eternity, I finally heard the familiar bell on Aussie's collar. Will and Aussie were on their way back home.

As Will came up the driveway, I saw him seeing me. I was standing at the top of the steps gleaming. There was a smile plastered on my face so big and bright it lit up the dark mountain sky. He knew. I was pregnant at last.

Nearly eight months of trying, strategizing, thinking about nothing else but how to conceive to be pregnant, and my miracle had finally occurred. The irony is this: The one month I wasn't focusing on getting pregnant, the one month I took conception as a second concern, this was the month I got pregnant.

The month my mother died was the month Will and I conceived.

Realizing that, I heard the dreadful whisper again. The horrid question I had the month prior was suddenly burned back into my mind like a tattoo. "Would you trade your mother's life to be pregnant?"

Had I answered? Did I unknowingly cut a deal? Was my mother gone because I chose having a baby over her life? Did my longing to be pregnant have more power than my love to save her? This would haunt me more than I realized at the time. The voice posed the question, and then accused and condemned. The joy of being pregnant was sucked out of me and replaced with a horrible selfish guilt.

The next morning, I had to get on a plane for the leadership retreat. Will and I skipped the excitement and celebration that I had hoped we would share. My emotions were all over the place. I was reserved on the outside, but inside I vacillated between elation and grief. I missed my mother terribly, and I felt immense guilt for wanting to be happy about my pregnancy. I wanted to tell her, to see the look on her face when I shared the blessed news with her. I had so many questions I wanted to ask her. I wanted to go shopping with her. I wanted her to tell me everything was going to be all right. But I couldn't. I couldn't do any of that. I had no mother to run to. I was all alone, torn between my joy, anger, and guilt.

CHAPTER TWO

Omens Of Fear And Guilt

"The minute you settle for less than you deserve,
you get even less than you settled for."

-Maureen Dowd

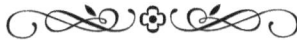

Aside from the emotional pain of grief and guilt I felt due to the loss of my mom (which I hid quite well, even from myself), my pregnancy with Zackery was perfect. There were no complications, and we were both healthy and growing. I loved knowing there was a little being inside me. I felt happy and beautiful. By the time I was able to feel him kicking and moving around, my favorite thing to do was to come home from work, sit on the couch, pull my shirt up, and watch my belly move in beautiful, wondrous waves.

I have always tried to live my life as naturally as possible, and so I wanted to give birth without painkillers. However, I did not want a home birth: hospitals have always felt safe to me. Will told me he would support any decision I made, and so I chose to work with a doula—a birth coach who would help train me for childbirth and guide me through the process. We settled on the

HypnoBirthing® method, which uses deep breathing, relaxation, and visualization techniques to reduce the fear and tension of giving birth, thus helping to reduce the pain.

Zackery Gendebien Zimmer was born naturally at 9:17 p.m. on September 15, 2007. He was 7 pounds 7 ounces, 19-1/2 inches long, and the most perfect little angel I had ever laid eyes on. I was flooded with love, pride, and even shock that Will and I now had this little beautiful baby. We had waited so long to meet him and now here he was, nestled in my arms as I gently stroked his soft, pure, delicate skin. Nothing else in the world mattered. That first night, Will held his son all night long, sleeping sitting up in a chair with Zack on a pillow. We both felt absolutely blissful. We were a family!

The birth was easy and beautiful (though painful), and everybody told me that it was one of the best they'd seen any mom do. But I knew it wasn't perfect. "Next time I'll do better," I told myself. I knew it was possible to do better because I had read all about it. Not being totally flawless made me just a little irritated and disappointed, but it didn't matter; we were planning to have another baby in two years. I'd fix it next time!

When we had walked into the hospital for Zackery's birth, I had been wearing flip-flops. When we left two days later, it was snowing. Winter had arrived early in our mountain town, and it would turn out to be a long one that would bury us in waist-deep snowdrifts for months. That winter would be a very difficult one for our new family.

My father made the four-hour drive up to meet Zackery and help Will and I bring him home from the hospital. He was wonderful support, helping Will change diapers, bringing me water and food, and running back and forth to buy pacifiers, wipes, and other random baby necessities.

At one point, dad came into my room to get Zackery after I had just finished nursing him, and he noticed I was crying.

"What's the matter?" he asked.

"I don't know," I answered.

He came over and hugged me, saying it was okay to cry, that it was normal, and I didn't have to have a reason. He was one of the first to give me permission to cry for no reason. It felt so good to have somebody accept my emotions without rationalizing them, and it still does.

There is more than one way to parent and take care of a child, but back then, I didn't think so. I had read the books and was sure there was one correct way of doing things—and I was so focused on this idea that I was horrified to make a mistake. What if Zackery started crying and I couldn't get him to stop? What if I changed the diaper wrong and hurt him or made a mess? The possibilities had total control over me. It wasn't that I couldn't physically do any of those things; for some reason, I felt that I didn't know how. Meanwhile, Will could take it all in stride. He was the one who could make Zack stop crying, who could handle a messy diaper change—anything that was freaking me out, Will handled with complete confidence.

Reclaim the Joy of Motherhood

For the first several weeks, maybe even a month, I don't think I ever changed a diaper. Will did everything. He cleaned Zackery's umbilical cord, swaddled him, brought him to me and took him from me for feedings, and held him when he cried (which he did a lot). Will even got up with me every single time Zackery needed feeding in the middle of the night, without fail. I was scared to be alone with Zack. It got so bad that I would only let Will leave the house once Zack was asleep, and I would make sure he would return before Zack awoke—which was difficult because Zack did not sleep well for long periods of time without being held or rocked. I didn't believe I could comfort our baby the way Will did. I was afraid to try because I was afraid I would do something wrong. I loved Zackery so deeply, but I was overwhelmed with anxiety. Without Will, I don't know what I would have done.

For the first three months, Will and I were both home with Zackery. Will had left his job several months before, but the economy was starting to take a nosedive and it was proving really difficult to find new work. I, on the other hand, had a job and didn't want to go.

When I had co-founded my architecture firm, my partner and I thought it would be a chance to do glamorous and fulfilling work. We soon found out that this wasn't always the case. We had a few custom projects, especially in the first year or two, for creative, open, willing, and trusting clients. But as our firm grew and needed more stability, we took on more dry, boring work: the bread-and-butter tasks that provided income without inspiration. Even with those, we had drafters to do the drawing, while we as business owners had to focus on the day-to-day work of running the office. My dream of architecture was to create unique, sustainable, inspiring, and beautifully composed buildings. Little by little, that dream was obscured and I lost my passion for my work.

My architecture partner was a great guy whose wife was an obstetrics RN, so he totally understood when I wanted to take eight weeks off for maternity leave—and he was even understanding when the eight weeks were up and I told him I needed more time. I stayed home another month, until Zackery was three months old. It was definitely time for me to go back to work. But even though it was what we had all talked about and planned, I just wasn't ready.

I really didn't have a choice, though. With Will out of work, I needed to be the breadwinner for our new little family. I started slowly with just eight hours a week and gradually increased it until finally, after six months, I was back at work four days for thirty hours a week. It was not full-time compared to corporate America, but it was all the time I could give. Will helped to make up the difference by taking a seasonal job doing snow removal, getting up at three in the morning to work exhausting hours on the mountain.

At this point, our baby books told us that Zackery should be sleeping through the night. It seemed logical that we could start going back to work, but something was wrong. Zackery was gassy and having digestive problems. He was always fussy and

19

wouldn't sleep for more than a few hours at a time. Eventually, we found out that he had food sensitivities—but in those first months, all we could do was hold him, rock him, and lavish him with love. We were both up throughout the night, and we were getting worn out.

If my name hadn't been on the door, I don't think I would have gone back to work at all. I dreaded every morning, crying as I got in my car and drove the short eight minutes to my office. I was not only exhausted and mentally uncertain, but despite my fear of independently taking care of Zackery, I was jealous of Will getting to be with him. I enjoyed having my own business, but it was no longer enough. Sometimes I started to resent myself for ever wanting a successful career.

I had wanted to breastfeed Zackery until he turned one, because that was what a perfect mom would do. I loved it, too: loved bonding with him, loved having him fall asleep on me in perfect bliss. I often slept in my rocking chair afterward, with him on my lap. But pretty soon, we discovered that his food sensitivities were related to what I was eating. I had to restrict my diet so his stomach wouldn't act up. Living on just chicken breast, avocado, and rice—not to mention pumping at work—I started to see my milk supply dropping, and eventually it stopped. I was so disappointed in myself. I really believed I should be able to do everything! I fell short of the one-year goal by over six months. Realistically, Zackery was happy and healthy and starting to eat real food, but I still felt like I had let him and myself down.

Will was (and still is) an amazing dad, and we both found glimpses of joy in watching Zackery grow and learn new things. I took a billion pictures of our happy baby; we brought him to music class and the local "baby and me" class to sing, learn, and make new friends. But between me and Will, things were getting to be difficult. I had never really opened up again after my mom's death, and the emotional distance between us was making it hard to act as a team. Add to that our mounting stress over work and money, even Zackery's beautiful face couldn't always cheer us up.

When Will and I had first planned our family, we'd figured on a second baby two years after Zack. But when we found out how difficult it was to have just one, we decided to wait a little longer. We also wanted to lessen the pressure of getting pregnant right away—and I was preoccupied with the idea of having a spring baby. The dark, cold winter months had been extremely isolating and lonely. I didn't want to go through that again with another newborn. By having my baby in the springtime, I hoped the long, warm days would help stave off the loneliness and discord I had felt during the months when Zack and I had been stuck in the house under eight feet of snow.

We started trying again when Zackery was a year and a half old. We wanted a girl, a sister for our darling boy. I believed I could control the gender of our baby through timing sex very precisely prior to ovulation. Was this possible? I was confident that it would work, and for a few months we tried—only to be disappointed. I had given myself a couple of months' cushion to get pregnant, but I also knew that if I truly wanted a spring baby then I had to conceive in the summer. And after four months of trying, I was feeling the same old disappointment. Summer would soon be over and the window of opportunity to have a spring baby was rapidly closing.

And then it happened! We got pregnant again, a little later than planned, but still soon enough that our new baby would come before high summer. It was to be a second boy, not a girl like we had hoped—but ultimately, we realized that was actually a good thing. In fact, now I am sure that I'm at my best as a mother to boys (and it doesn't hurt that my sons can share clothes and toys). Later, I came to realize that this baby, who we decided to call Brayden, was a blessing in more ways than one. Brayden's love would one day save me.

My pregnancy with Brayden was good, as it had been with Zackery. I was glowing with excitement and the knowledge of another little angel growing inside me. It was what I loved the most about having children: the life inside me. I was good at being pregnant.

I'm not sure if it was just because I was more aware of my body the second time around, but physically my pregnancy symptoms were more pronounced. I was much more nauseous—for the entire first trimester—and actually lost weight. My back hurt more, and my sciatica kept me from staying in any one position for more than ten minutes at a time. I didn't sleep as well and was completely engulfed in fatigue. But no matter how much it seemed my body was hurting, warning me perhaps that I needed to take better care, I was in love with being pregnant once again.

At thirty-four weeks—six weeks before Brayden would be "full term"—I started having contractions. These weren't just random Braxton Hicks "practice" contractions. They were real. Hard, tight and every ten minutes—like clockwork. They went on for an hour before I decided, that yes, this was happening. I told Will, and we immediately called our doula, Marlena.

She got to our house within fifteen minutes, during which time I gathered my purse, my cell phone and my water bottle, but couldn't really gather the reality of what was happening. Marlena told us that the doctor would try to stop the contractions, but that there was a chance Brayden would be born tonight.

We had no one to come over and stay at the house while Zackery slept, so Will had to stay home. As Marlena helped me walk down the steps and get into her car, I realized that Will was left to watch as his wife and unborn baby were departing. We were not going to be together. Then it hit me, and I got really scared.

If Brayden had been born that night, I know we all would have survived it—but it would have been devastating for both Will and I to not be together, to not have things go as we planned. I was so glad that Marlena was with me, to keep my mind off of the potential possibility of having a preemie. Thankfully, the doctor was able to stop my contractions, but my stress level was through the roof. The doctor put me on restricted activity, and I obeyed. All I wanted to do was hold on to my healthy pregnancy for at least another three weeks.

Reclaim the Joy of Motherhood

Just like Zackery, Brayden was born at thirty-eight weeks. At 11:58 p.m., on June 27, 2010, I again gave birth naturally through HypnoBirthing® to a healthy, 7-pound, 11-ounce, 19-inch baby boy: Brayden Ivanocko Zimmer. Giving birth was one of the most painful things I have ever experienced in my entire life, but it was also the most breathtaking, miraculous, and wonderful. When the nurse placed Brayden on my chest, both of us naked, I knew right then and there that our family was complete. But even then, in the back of my mind, I was a little disappointed. I had been determined to have the perfect birth experience, and although Brayden's birth was even better than Zackery's, there were a few small instances where I felt I could've pushed through and focused more, or used my HypnoBirthing training and practice just a little more to have done better.

The next morning, my father again made the relatively short trip up to meet his second grandson, picking up Zackery from the babysitter so he could see his new little baby brother for the first time. It brought me such joy to see Zack holding Brayden in his lap. At first he was timid and afraid to come near our new baby, but once he got a little more comfortable, Zackery's tenderness and loving kindness shone through. I was so happy, in that moment, for the beautiful family that Will and I had created.

Will, Brayden, and I stayed in the hospital three nights, one night longer than I had with Zackery. Part of me felt guilty for not coming home to be with Zack right away, but I knew that he was in good hands with my father, the babysitter, the neighbors, and his daycare. Brayden and I were having difficulty with his latch for breastfeeding, and I was eager and receptive to having the extra help, support, and guidance of the amazing nursing staff.

I think part of me was also starting to feel scared about taking our beloved Brayden home. I was beginning to have thoughts of inadequacy and doubted my decisions of how to care for him. I knew I had felt that way before with Zackery, nearly three years prior, and I knew I would have to face those fears.

CHAPTER THREE

Full-Time Architect To Full-Time Mom

*"Change, like sunshine, can be a friend or a foe,
a blessing or a curse, a dawn or a dusk"*

-William Arthur Ward

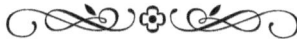

Three weeks before Brayden joined our family, I had my very last day as principal architect and owner of my own business. June 1st was my last day of work—my last day sitting at my desk reviewing plans, talking to contractors, meeting with clients, approving timesheets, and signing checks. It was my last day as an architect and the first day of the next chapter in my life, entitled "motherhood."

I couldn't have left my career at a better time. The economy had crashed, and our business was not as profitable as it had been in prior years. My business partner and I had been forced to downsize and lay off our employees, and the bulk of our clients had put their projects on hold or canceled them altogether. We went a year without paying ourselves, literally to keep the doors open and the lights on.

Things were difficult financially at home, too. Thanks to the crash, we were upside down on our house, and our savings were running out. It was time for a change. Will had embarked on a new career in insurance, and was actively working—not for much money at first, but we knew it would be profitable in the long run. Meanwhile, my desire to be home with my boys was overwhelming. It felt like the right thing to support Will's career and our growing family, and it felt right to stay at home. I was a mom now, and that was just more important to me than architecture.

The reality of leaving work was bittersweet: I was giving up the career I had worked so long and hard to have. I felt guilty leaving my business partner, particularly at a time when our business was no longer flourishing. At the same time, deep down inside I felt relief. My heart wasn't in it anymore. I had always loved being an architect, but that didn't mean I loved having to go to work every day. I had lost my passion and needed to release myself from what felt more like an obligation than a purpose.

So here I was, at home with a newborn baby, feeling like a brand new mom for the first time. Yes, Brayden was my second, but it was the first time I was the at-home parent. It was the first time I was responsible and in charge: with Will working, I had to do the bulk of the diaper changes, the tummy time, the baths, and the swaddling. Zackery was in daycare four days a week; during the day it was just me and Brayden. He ate, he pooped, he slept, just like any newborn would and should do. But it wasn't that easy. It should have been, but it wasn't.

Along with the consistent challenge of a proper latch (which, as any mother who has tried breastfeeding knows, is important not only for your milk supply and prevention of clogged ducts, but also for the prevention of nipple pain), Brayden and I both fought an on-and-off battle with thrush for two and a half months.

It got so bad that every time I had to nurse Brayden I would break down and cry in anticipation of the pain. The pinching of Brayden's latch, which by that time had already become his habit, was excruciating. It wouldn't always last the entire feeding; sometimes I was able to correct him, but it always started out with me wincing in agony, begging him to open wider.

Add to that the other side effects of the thrush—my itching, burning nipple irritation, and Brayden's extreme diaper rash— and it's no wonder I had people telling me to stop breastfeeding. But I wouldn't. I wouldn't give up or give in. I know there are women who choose not to or simply cannot breastfeed, and I openly support each individual's choice, but for me, breastfeeding was important. Brayden was my baby and I was going to feed him, the way I had imagined I would, the way I believed was the most natural and beneficial, even if it meant becoming a martyr.

Apparently, my life shows no sympathy for irony, and everything does happen for a reason. In the past, whenever anybody asked me, "What do you do?" I had an easy answer: "I'm an architect." Everybody knew what that meant, and most people were impressed. It was something that really set me apart. Now I was entering a new and less structured role, and I was losing part of my identity. If I wasn't an architect, who was I? If I was going to give up my career for motherhood, I felt I would have to become the perfect mom.

Reclaim the Joy of Motherhood

Of course that was my own perception, part of my lifelong tendency to hold myself to an unreal standard. "Perfect mom"— what is that? It would be years before I could finally understand what an amazing accomplishment it is to be a good mother: to bring life into the world and nurture it. Eventually, I would learn that happiness is enough, that there are many different ways to get there, and that motherhood is its own goal. But now, I was approaching it like an architect would: with a strict set of guidelines that needed to be met in order to achieve success. The painful breastfeeding, in my mind, was a price worth paying for my baby's future. And especially after I had "failed" at nursing Zackery for a full year, I was absolutely determined to get it right this time.

Eventually, after multiple creams, ointments, diet restrictions, and pills (prescription and not), I found a homeopathic remedy that worked: Genitian Violet. It turned my breasts and Brayden's mouth purple, and I felt quite silly and uncomfortably bashful walking around my house with no shirt or bra, but thankfully it worked. Brayden's crankiness (a symptom of thrush) subsided, and "normal" breastfeeding resumed.

With Brayden, my goal again was to breastfeed for one year. Breastfeeding with Brayden was different than with Zackery. Because I wasn't working, I didn't need to have such a strict, by-the-book schedule as I had followed with Zackery. There were pros and cons to this: Nursing could take fifteen minutes or forty-five, and Brayden could get hungry again after four hours or after only two (sometimes even less). It was exhausting and depleting,

30

and it was hard to just let go, but in my heart it felt like the right thing to do. So I did it. I wanted to be present with Brayden, and he taught me that it was okay. Over time, we began working together as a team, and it started getting easier for us both.

I was taking other positive steps, too. I had wanted a spring baby, partly so that I would feel more inclined to get out of the house during Brayden's infancy: enjoying the sunshine, fresh air, and pine trees in the beautiful, postcard-like Sierra Nevada mountains. I hadn't been able to do that during the heavy snows when Zackery was small, and I believed the isolation had been a big contributor to my "Baby Blues" with him. With Brayden, the weather was cooperative, and just as I'd planned, I made a concerted effort to get us both out of the house. We went on errands to the grocery store, on walks, and to the yoga-and-baby class. I also went consistently to breastfeeding class (more of a support group run by the local lactation consultant) and the baby-and-me group every week. I forced myself to be social and active. I was not going to get depressed this time!

"I am a strong woman," I kept telling myself, and I was feeling good about how much I was actually out and about with Brayden, all on my own. I felt good about being confident in caring for him, and especially proud of being able to put him to sleep in his crib, all on my own. I was proactively heading down a happy path; sadness could kiss my butt goodbye.

I was tired, as I assumed anybody who hadn't slept well in years would be. To me, the fatigue felt normal. I thought this was how I was supposed to be feeling. It didn't even cross my mind that I should be feeling any differently, or that the new moms around me weren't as tired as I was. When I shed tears for no particular reason, I believed it was just lack of sleep. If I could just get some consistent rest, I thought, I would feel better.

At times, I thought about my own mother, and what it would have been like to have her presence in our lives. I missed her. I missed hearing her voice, smelling the soft scent of her perfume, and watching her smile break into giggles of bubbling laughter. What hurt the most, however, was not having her here to meet her grandsons. She would never be able to hold them. They would never be able to sit in her lap while she read a bedtime story. They would never be able to hold her hand or feel her nurturing wisdom. I missed my mother, as much for myself as for my sons.

Also, at times, I was jealous of my friends who had their own moms to help with their babies. What would it be like, I wondered, to have that companionship and guidance? When I didn't know what to do, wouldn't it have been wonderful to call up my mom and ask for advice? Her absence was a void that nobody else could fill. Will's mother lived far away, in Pennsylvania, and though she was supportive and kind—she'd even flown out for Zackery's baby shower—it wasn't the same as having my own mom on the other end of the phone line. Later, I would come to understand that I was still grieving the loss of my mother, even years later. But at the time, it was something that was out of my control and not worth crying over. So, aside from the occasional inexplicable fountain of tears, I shut my feelings away behind a locked door.

In September, when Brayden was just a couple of months old, there was a new door to close: my old architectural office was shutting down. My partner, no longer able to bear the weight of the struggling business, had found a job out of town. We discussed it at length, and decided the time had come to close the business. And although I was no longer working, I was still technically an officer of the corporation. My finances—our family's finances—were tied to this business. What had been my life's purpose, then an obligation, and finally a phase to leave behind, was now an unwanted burden.

Will and I were out of money. We were not surviving on Will's small income, especially with payments on a house that was worth less than what we owed. We now needed to find a way to pay off the business loans. With no other option, we were forced to file for personal bankruptcy. All we had was our upside down house and our two boys (Zackery barely three years old, and Brayden about to be just three months old).

Because my business partner had moved to start his new job, it fell to me to finalize the closing of our office. So one day in the yellow light of September, I went back to oversee the demolition of a dream.

With Brayden in his infant carrier, I stepped up to the front door where I had once felt passion and pride to see my name etched in the clear glass. I put the key into the lock and turned, feeling it release with a dull click. I pushed, opening the door just enough for Brayden and I to fit through. We stepped inside to see what was left of my years of hard work.

The office was devoid of people, but it was far from empty. There were still stacks of boxes filled with old client drawings and accounting files; office furniture and equipment; and so many memories of what I had helped to build, now being demolished and discarded.

I was overwhelmed. How would I possibly be able to get rid of all this stuff? Not only was it physically too much for me to move on my own, but mentally it was demoralizing. Here I was, standing in the middle of what I thought I had already left behind—but it was still here, in shambles, and I was going to have to deal with it. This time, there was no option to just move on without a backward glance. I was going to have to say a final goodbye to my business, to seven years of hard work, seven years of my life. And I was going to have to do it piece by piece.

Calling upon the determination my mother had once told me she always saw in me, I set out to get it done. The next few weeks were spent in that dusty, silent office that had once thrummed with the beat of my heart. As always, Will gave me his unconditional support and plenty of physical help. Box by box, drawing by drawing, we made every trace of that life disappear. On October 1st, I handed back the keys to a vacant space. It was ready for someone else's dreams.

I felt so tired. All my determination, all the things I had set my mind to in life—would they all turn out this way? I was lost in a maze of failure. Everywhere I looked, something was going wrong. My mother was gone, we had no money, my business had failed, and I was nowhere near the unrealistic goal of becoming a perfect mom. My boys (all three of them) were a guiding light that kept me going: When I got out of bed in the mornings, it was because I knew they needed me and that, even in some small way, I might be able to do something good to make their lives better. But it all felt hopeless in the end. I couldn't have told you what difference it would make, in the long run, whether I got out of bed or not. Nothing seemed clear anymore, and it was harder and harder to care.

CHAPTER FOUR

What's Happening to Me?

"When you're lost in those woods, it sometimes takes you a while to realize that you are lost. For the longest time, you can convince yourself that you've just wandered off the path, that you'll find your way back to the trailhead any moment now. Then night falls again and again, and you still have no idea where you are, and it's time to admit that you have bewildered yourself so far off the path that you don't even know from which direction the sun rises anymore."

-Elizabeth Gilbert

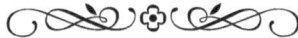

***

It's three o'clock in the morning. My eyes are barely peeled open, heavy and achy from lack of sleep. I hear Brayden, just four months old, fussing in his crib at the foot of our bed. It takes every iota of energy in my body, every speck of strength I can muster, to drag myself from the depths of my interrupted slumber to the chair three feet away. I am so tired. All I want to do is sleep forever. I want to sleep peaceful and warm, tucked into my sanctuary. I don't want to ever worry about the next time I have to get up, or the next time I have to do anything. I just want to sleep—forever.

Reclaim the Joy of Motherhood

*My husband tenderly picks up Brayden. In the quiet darkness, with
only a tiny ray of light from the green, red, and yellow elephant-safari
nightlight, he changes our baby's tiny little diaper. By now, I have made
the trek to my spot: the soft, sage green, reclining rocking chair. I'm
situated as perfectly as I can be, with the soles of my slippered feet on the
slanted wooden footrest and the soft boppy pillow positioned purposefully
on my lap waiting to nestle my newborn. With cold hands, I gently slip
open my nursing nightgown, unclip my bra, remove the cotton breast
pad and place it carefully next to my water bottle on the makeshift table
next to me.*

*I reach my arms out to take Brayden from Will, now standing in front
of me, ready for our choreographed handoff. As I cradle Brayden to my
breast, I feel the delicate weight of a blanket lovingly being placed over
my legs, shoulders, and Brayden's precious little body, leaving only
his head and my breast exposed to the chilly night air. For a moment,
everything seems fine, beautiful like a flawlessly performed dance under a
moonlit sky.*

*And then it hits: a sharp pain in my chest, so startling it steals my
breath. The shake throughout my body even startles Brayden. For a split
second, he removes his soft lips from my breast. What is happening to
me? I ask myself. I am frightened, almost paralyzed. Is it my heart? Am I
having a heart attack?*

*The piercing sharpness quickly retreats into a persistent dull ball
of pressure. I am uncomfortable and scared, but I continue to nurse
Brayden without making a sound. Instead of calling out for help, I
quietly plead with my body to make the pain stop. I beg for relief, but*

*there is none. The only thing that helps me mentally fight this horror
is the innocent little baby I have nestled in my arms. I forge on. I am a
strong woman. In spite of the pain, I am determined to nurse my son.
Gazing down at him, I make him my only priority.*

*Once Brayden is sound asleep with a full little tummy and the security
of a tight swaddle, I place him gently in his crib. With my hand over my
heart, I make my way back to my side of the bed and crawl in. The pain
is still there, made brighter and more threatening by my mounting fear. I
remain silent. A tear rolls down my cheek, and I slowly drift off to sleep.*

As it too often did, the light of morning came quickly. I resented
it. I had no choice but to participate in the routine of the day: get
out of bed, nurse Brayden, dress him, get him settled on the floor
or in the bouncy chair or swing, fix myself something to eat, fill
my water bottle, help Will get Zackery ready for daycare. These
tasks were so difficult for me, and took so much energy to do, that
I didn't even bother brushing my teeth, getting myself dressed, or
even sometimes taking a shower. Those last three didn't happen
very often these days. Usually, I stayed in my pajamas (which
typically consisted of yoga pants, a nursing tank top, and a zip-
front sweatshirt) for days at a time. It was too much effort to
change my clothes, let alone take a shower. Will had to force me to
shower—not physically, but by telling me over and over to "just
go take a shower" until finally I mustered up the energy (drawing
upon his motivation) to give myself the luxury of standing under
the warm water and getting clean. I always felt better after the
shower—refreshed and a tiny bit re-energized—but it never
lasted, and I usually fell straight back into my rut and another set
of unwashed clothes.

Reclaim the Joy of Motherhood

Mornings were hard, but at least I had Will there to help me. Once he took Zackery to daycare, leaving me with only Brayden to care for, things actually got worse. When Will was gone, it was all me. I had to rely on my own decisions: when to nurse Brayden, when to change him, and when to put him down to sleep. What if he cried or had a terribly dirty diaper, or what if he wouldn't sleep? What if he wouldn't latch properly during nursing, or what if my milk wasn't enough for him? What if he wasn't happy? What if I dropped him or forgot about him? What if he started crying during the thirty seconds I left to go to the bathroom? What if I shook him? What if I pushed him? What if I hurt him? What if those "what-ifs" didn't stop? What on earth would I do?

Those were the thoughts that ran through my head: thoughts of inadequacy when it came to caring for my baby. Scary thoughts of things that could go wrong; although they were the last things I would ever actually want to do to my baby, they were thoughts I couldn't get rid of. These thoughts clouded my mind all day long, always there prodding at me. Winter had come again, and the short days kept me and Brayden indoors with my ever-growing list of worries and tasks.

I held fast to my daily routine: nursing Brayden, changing him, engaging and stimulating his growing mind (with books, toys, and tummy time, or just talking to him or taking him for a walk down the street), putting him down for naps. I repeated this pattern two, three, or four times during the day; then I had to pick up Zackery from daycare, give him dinner, and figure out something to eat for myself. Sometimes Will would be home for dinner (and sometimes he even would be able to pick up Zackery, which was a big relief for me), but my daily schedule was dependent primarily upon Brayden's schedule, which seemed to change constantly. Add bath nights, grocery shopping, doctor appointments, breastfeeding class, and baby-and-me class, and it became overwhelming. I needed those activities to get me and Brayden out of the house, but I dreaded them nonetheless.

To the outside world, to my husband, and even to myself at times, my life seemed simple: a baby and his mother—someone to care for him, to nurture him, to feed him, to hold him, to love him. But it wasn't simple. It wasn't simple at all!

Caring for Brayden correctly was foremost in my mind. I second-guessed and questioned myself all the time. I constantly felt like I was doing something wrong. My poor mothering was the imaginary reason for my nursing pain, our two-and-a-half-month battle with thrush, Brayden's trouble sleeping through the night, and on and on. I believed everything that was going wrong was my fault, that I wasn't good enough. What if I wasn't?

What if the "what-if" thoughts took over and I wouldn't be strong enough to make the right decision? I felt like I didn't know who I was anymore. This wasn't me, but I didn't know who I should be either.

The morning after my frightening chest pains, the sharp sensation had disappeared, but the feeling was burned into my brain as clear as anything I had ever seen or felt. Once I put Brayden in his crib, happily taking his morning nap, I had a chance to sit down on the couch with my laptop and search for answers. I clicked on the little icon at the bottom left corner of the screen and waited for the browser to appear. The cursor flashed an invitation into the infinite realm of the World Wide Web. I took a deep breath, and with certainty, typed in the words "heart attack in women."

The search results appeared so matter-of-factly. One by one, I buried myself in the words of each article, each statistic, and each story. Unexpectedly, I realized with relief that the pain I had experienced mere hours before was not, in fact, a heart attack. Yes, I had felt the shaking, the fear and anxiety, the absolutely crippling pain in my chest. But I was still alive.

Okay… so what is happening to me? My mind traveled through a weaving, thorn-filled path of possible alternatives, knowing quite well the probable answer to my earlier question. I was in denial of the obvious alternative. From the depths of my soul, I knew what most likely caused my monstrous episode. I was terrified to even think about it, let alone acknowledge or accept it, but I had no choice.

I cleared the words "heart attack in women" and, with shaking fingers, replaced them with "Postpartum Depression"—two words I had never imagined would mean anything to me. It seemed unreal, impossible, and debilitating. Almost in tears, I scrolled through the findings.

"...but you may not know that depression can be associated with many physical symptoms, too. In fact, many people with depression..."

"...postpartum depression symptoms can include physical ones like headaches and nausea..."

"...it is common to develop physical symptoms such as headaches, palpitations, chest pains, and general aches. Some people consult a..."

I hesitated, scared to commit to any entry. I knew I didn't have much more time before Brayden would wake, and I would need to be physically and mentally up to the task of taking care of him. Once again, with a deep breath, I selected a heading that I hoped would be the least destructive to my current fragile state of mind...

...and...

...click!

What I found shocked me.

"Many women have the Baby Blues after childbirth. If you have the baby blues, you may have mood swings, feel sad, anxious or overwhelmed, have crying spells, lose your appetite, or have trouble sleeping. The baby blues often go away within a few days or a week.... The symptoms of postpartum depression last longer and are more severe. You may also feel hopeless and worthless, and lose interest in the baby. You may have thoughts of hurting yourself or the baby."[1]

In a daze, I clicked another link.

"Most of us know about the emotional symptoms of depression. But you may not know that depression can be associated with many physical symptoms, too. Because these symptoms occur

43

with many conditions, many depressed people never get help, because they don't know that their physical symptoms might be caused by depression. A lot of doctors miss the symptoms, too. These physical symptoms aren't 'all in your head.' Depression can cause real changes in your body." [2]

It seemed surreal. I never knew that depression could cause physical symptoms. I had no idea. Continuing to read the article, I learned that depression can actually cause people to experience pain differently or more severely. Wow! This whole time I believed depression was purely a mental thing, something in the brain.

I didn't want to believe it, but I was reading about me! I had almost all the symptoms: headaches, backache, muscle and joint pain, chest pain, fatigue and exhaustion, sleeping problems, and change in appetite. I had it all. It was as if this website was my journal, describing what I was experiencing, in a way that until now I could not put into words. I had thought I was making it all up, but after reading this I knew, I knew it was real.

I was riddled with mixed emotions. I felt relieved that what I was experiencing could be identified and treated. Postpartum Depression was real and wasn't just a figment of my imagination. But knowing this didn't give me comfort or solace. In fact, I was frightened and shaking, perhaps more so now that reality was beginning to sink in.

I continued to read through my Internet searches, website after website:

"You may have Postpartum Depression if you have had a baby within the last 12 months and...you feel overwhelmed... guilty...you don't feel bonded to your baby...you are confused and scared...irritated or angry...you feel nothing...sadness... can't stop crying...hopeless...like a failure...in a fog...you know something is wrong." [3]

I read until tears clouded my vision and I could no longer see the words in front of me. I read until the facts were branded into my memory, flashing like neon warning signs.

I read until I heard Brayden's tiny whimpers as he awoke from his dreamland. I didn't know which was worse: having to snap back into my role as Brayden's mother, or being unable to escape what I had just learned. I could not hide from the truth: that the pains and horrors of my worst living nightmare were all symptoms of Postpartum Depression. Symptoms I never knew could take such a strong hold and reveal themselves in such ugly, cruel, mental and physical ways. If this was real, was it my new "normal?"

The next few hours were a blur. I drifted in and out of caring for Brayden. I was filled with uncertainty, worry, guilt, and nervousness. I was anxious. I wrestled with my brain to accept or not accept the facts I had just learned. I didn't want to believe any of it. I didn't want to feel this way. I had worked very hard to prevent getting Postpartum Depression. I had been proactive and strong. This was NOT fair! This was NOT me! This could NOT be my fate! This was simply WRONG!

Reclaim the Joy of Motherhood

The day lingered on into the night and I stopped paying attention to the passage of time, until I had no idea what day it was and had no desire to even find out. I didn't care. I didn't care about anything. I still kept silent, not saying a word to Will or anyone. It was my little secret. If I didn't say it out loud, no one would know and then maybe it wouldn't be true. Words would give it life and I didn't want to do that. I wanted it to go away. I tried desperately to erase the visions of judgment, to quiet the voices inside telling me that I was broken and that this was my fault. The voices telling me that I didn't deserve to be a mother, that I was weak, sad, and worthless. I tried to escape my own mind but nothing worked.

I wanted to feel, feel anything at all, but I didn't. I couldn't. I tried to persuade myself to experience joy and love. I had this wonderful, precious little bundle of joy—a true living miracle—but I couldn't engage. I didn't know how. I wasn't happy. I wasn't anything except a lifeless body going through motions that had no meaning to me. I was literally drained and had no energy. My plug into life had short-circuited and was beyond repair. I felt myself spiraling downward, faster and faster, to where no one could see me. I could barely see myself.

But I had this baby, Brayden. He saw me… and he wouldn't take his eyes off of me.

CHAPTER FIVE

What's Happening to You?

"Even though you may want to move forward in your life, you may have one foot on the brakes. In order to be free, we must learn how to let go. Release the hurt. Release the fear. Refuse to entertain your old pain. The energy it takes to hang onto the past is holding you back from a new life. What is it you would let go of today?"

- Mary Manin Morrissey

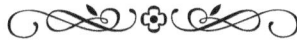

It took me over a year to write that last chapter. When I started writing, it was more of a journal. Several months had passed since that frightening night. I was getting treatment for my Postpartum Depression, and it was paying off. I had been on medication for some time, and was looking forward to not needing it anymore. Will was working, Zackery was in preschool three days a week, and Brayden was home with me (where I finally felt able to care for him without becoming overwhelmed). Our sons were growing up beautifully, our financial position had stabilized, and I was finally starting to feel like myself again: a strong, intelligent woman who could do anything I set my mind to. I had set my mind to writing my story, but it was extremely difficult to go back to that place again and again. I'd be at the library or the coffee shop, and I'd write for an hour or half an hour, and that would be it; I couldn't go further. It was too emotionally painful.

But because I am who I am, I needed a purpose. And that purpose, for me, was YOU. Over time, I discovered that my motivation to write this book was no longer about me, but about the other women like me, out there somewhere, who were going through the same thing all alone. I felt that, if I could get this story out, maybe another new mom would read it and be able to get help. That gave me hope—YOU gave me hope—to keep writing and finish it. It has been the most healing thing I've experienced, and for that I thank you, whoever you are.

In this chapter, I will give you the definitions you need to understand what Postpartum Depression really is. I'm also going to ask some questions, and I want you to be completely honest. This is a safe place. Write your answers here on the pages—and then you can close this book and hide it, lock it in a box, do whatever you need to do to feel protected with the truth here. Or, you can share it. Maybe that will happen later. For right now, it is just you, me, some hard questions, and a few even harder facts.

The Edinburgh Postnatal Depression Scale [4]

The following questions make up the Edinburgh Postnatal Depression Scale. It's the most commonly used tool to screen for potential PPD.

Edinburgh Postnatal Depression Scale (EPDS)

Name: _____

Address: _____

Your Date of Birth: _____

Baby's Date of Birth: _____

Phone: _____

As you are pregnant or have recently had a baby, we would like to know how you are feeling. Please check the answer that comes closest to how you have felt IN THE PAST 7 DAYS, not just how you feel today.

Here is an example, already completed.

I have felt happy:

○   Yes, all the time

☑   Yes, most of the time

○   No, not very often

○   No, not at all

This would mean: "I have felt happy most of the time" during the past week. Please complete the other questions in the same way.

In the past 7 days:

1. I have been able to laugh and see the funny side of things.

○ As much as I always could

○ Not quite so much now

○ Definitely not so much now

○ Not at all

2. I have looked forward with enjoyment to things.

○ As much as I ever did

○ Rather less than I used to

○ Definitely less than I used to

○ Hardly at all

3. *I have blamed myself unnecessarily when things went wrong.

○ Yes, most of the time

○ Yes, some of the time

○ Not very often

○ No, never

4. I have been anxious or worried for no good reason.

○ No not at all

○ Hardly ever

○ Yes, sometimes

○ Yes, very often

5. *I have felt scared or panicky for no very good reason.

- ○ Yes, quite a lot
- ○ Yes, sometimes
- ○ No, not much
- ○ No, not at all

6. *Things have been getting on top of me.

- ○ Yes, most of the time I haven't been able to cope at all
- ○ Yes, sometimes I haven't been coping as well as usual
- ○ No, most of the time I have coped quite well
- ○ No, I have been coping as well as ever

7. *I have been so unhappy that I have had difficulty sleeping.

- ○ Yes, most of the time
- ○ Yes, sometimes
- ○ Not very often
- ○ No, not at all

8. *I have felt sad or miserable.

- ○ Yes, most of the time
- ○ Yes, sometimes
- ○ Not very often
- ○ No, not at all

9. *I have been so unhappy that I have been crying.

    ○ Yes, most of the time

    ○ Yes, quite often

    ○ Only occasionally

    ○ No, never

10. *The thought of harming myself has occurred to me.

    ○ Yes, quite often

    ○ Sometimes

    ○ Hardly ever

    ○ Never

Administered/Reviewed by _____

Date _____

Postpartum depression is the most common complication of childbearing. The 10-question Edinburgh Postnatal Depression Scale (EPDS) is a valuable and efficient way of identifying patients at risk for "perinatal" depression. The EPDS is easy to administer and has proven to be an effective screening tool.

Mothers who score above 13 are likely to be suffering from a depressive illness of varying severity. The EPDS score should not override clinical judgment. A careful clinical assessment should be carried out to confirm the diagnosis. The scale indicates how the mother has felt during the previous week. In doubtful cases it may be useful to repeat the tool after 2 weeks. The scale will not detect mothers with anxiety neuroses, phobias or personality disorders.

Scoring

QUESTIONS 1, 2, & 4 (without an *)

Are scored 0, 1, 2 or 3 with top box scored as 0 and the bottom box scored as 3.

QUESTIONS 3 , 5 - 10 (marked with an *)

Are reverse scored, with the top box scored as a 3 and the bottom box scored as 0.

Maximum score: 30

Possible Depression: 10 or greater

Always look at item 10 (suicidal thoughts)

Instructions for using the Edinburgh Postnatal Depression Scale:

1. The mother is asked to check the response that comes closest to how she has been feeling in the previous 7 days.

2. All the items must be completed.

3. Care should be taken to avoid the possibility of the mother discussing her answers with others. (Answers come from the mother or pregnant woman.)

4. The mother should complete the scale herself, unless she has limited English or has difficulty with reading.

Fill in your score: _____

Sources: [5,6]

What is Postpartum Depression?

The two things you need to understand about Postpartum Depression are that it is treatable, and that it is not anyone's fault. Not even yours.

According to the National Library of Medicine, Postpartum Depression is "moderate to severe depression in a woman after she has given birth. It may occur soon after delivery or up to a year later. Most of the time, it occurs within the first three months after delivery."[7] PPD is a temporary medical condition that, left untreated, can last up to a year or more, having significant negative effects on the relationship of the entire family. It is not anything that can be fully predicted and/or prevented, and it affects a surprising number of women.

The statistics are staggering. The research I uncovered just before my own diagnosis of Postpartum Depression stated that one in eight mothers suffer from PPD. Only a few years later, some sources claim that statistic has risen to one in seven women, and even up to one in five! Some researchers believe (and I tend to agree with them) that the percentage of reported cases has increased because women are becoming more aware of PPD and are seeking help. Who knows what the number of unreported cases is each year.

Women are still afraid to talk about Postpartum Depression, even to their doctors or care providers. Instead, they remain silent, like I did, and suffer alone without hope or help. If my efforts can make even the slightest difference they will be well worth it.

Postpartum Depression does not discriminate. It can happen to any woman, regardless of age, race, culture, social status, or income level. It can occur in women who have already had children, in women who have adopted, and even after miscarriage or stillbirth. Surprisingly, it can even occur in men, affecting up to ten percent of new fathers.

Baby Blues vs. PPD

Statistically, up to eighty percent of all new mothers experience some kind of mood-related symptoms during the first two weeks following childbirth.[10] Typically called the Baby Blues, these symptoms usually fade away on their own within the first two to six weeks, often within three weeks. When symptoms persist or worsen, becoming more severe and/or frequent, this is called Postpartum Depression (PPD).

Because it's so common for new moms to feel "off" or "blue," these feelings are usually considered to be fairly normal—for a little while. But if after several months, your friends and family are telling you to "just mommy up" or "stop worrying about everything," they might be missing the reality that you are dealing with something more serious.

It is important to remember that the signs of PPD do not always appear immediately after childbirth—sometimes not for several weeks or months after what would be the normal Baby Blues period. "While the Baby Blues often look similar to the early stages of Postpartum Depression, there exist vast differences between the two phenomena," says Valerie McManus, a social worker and psychotherapist. "A skilled practitioner could differentiate between the two, ensuring an expedited response and treatment plan when postpartum depression is present." Unfortunately for most of us, our current medical system does not place enough importance on screening for these conditions. It is important for you to be aware of what is going on in your own body, your own mind.

Gauging Your Symptoms

When you're experiencing PPD, you might find it difficult to function well, or to bond with your baby. Some women, like I did, fear they will harm themselves or endanger their baby. This belief can become very real, which is why it is so important to talk to your doctor or care provider about these symptoms as soon as you notice them.

Here are some of PPD's most common symptoms. Next to each of these, put a number from 0 to 5, where 0 means you don't feel this symptom and 5 means you feel it very strongly.

____ Feelings of hopelessness, or helplessness

____ Feelings of worry or anxiety

____ Feelings of sadness or crying all the time

____ Feelings of guilt or shame

____ Irritability or mood swings

____ Lack of focus or difficulty concentrating

____ Fatigue or exhaustion

____ Trouble sleeping

_____ Changes in appetite

_____ Lack of interest in activities you would normally enjoy

_____ Feeling withdrawn or disconnected

_____ Headaches, backaches, or other body aches

_____ Problems doing everyday tasks at home or work

_____ Inability or lack of desire to care for your baby or yourself

_____ Negative feelings towards your baby

_____ Fear of being alone with your baby

_____ Thoughts of harming your baby, your other children, and/or yourself

_____ Thoughts of death or suicide

Is anything else going on that you feel is out of the ordinary, wrong, or "off?" Use this space to explain:

_____

_____

_____

_____

_____

_____

_____

_____

_____

_____

When you talk to your doctor or care provider, bring them this information. It can be incredibly hard to open up and describe what is happening. We will talk about that more in future chapters; you've already started the work by getting your feelings out on this page. Just by writing down the strength of your symptoms, you should already be seeing some new truths. The information on this page can also help a professional give you the best care.

When to Get Help

If you've made it this far, you probably know already that you should talk to somebody. In a few chapters, I'm going to help you do just that. But if you are ready now—and especially if you are thinking about hurting yourself or your baby—by all means, reach out to a doctor, a family member, a friend, an online message board—anyone.

If you're scared, confused, or don't feel like you're ready to make it "real" yet, I hope you will get in touch with me. I really did write this book for you, and I really am here to listen and be your friend. I understand where you are, because I've been on every single rung of the ladder. I would love nothing more than to talk with you and help make sense of it all.

Really, there is no reason why you should not talk to your doctor or care provider. You have not done anything wrong, what's happening is not rare, and it's not your fault. It's okay to say something if you just don't feel like yourself or you feel like something just isn't right. Don't be afraid to be open and honest about any changes you notice. It might not be anything, or it might be some form of Postpartum Depression, Postpartum Anxiety, or even Postpartum Psychosis. All of these illnesses are real, some are more common than others, and some more severe than others. The good news is that with the proper help, all can be treated.

Just remember, the sooner you seek help, the sooner you will begin to feel better.

What is Your Story?

There is no single cause for Postpartum Depression. There are no laboratory tests to diagnose it, yet it is the most common problem associated with childbirth. Early on, it was assumed that PPD was triggered by hormone changes in new mothers, or the complications of a traumatic birth, but that isn't necessarily the case. External circumstances also play a critical role, as they did for me.

I have no doubt that the combination of grief over my mother's death, anxiety over financial and work troubles for me and Will alike, and our sons' minor health challenges all contributed to my own PPD. Yours can be triggered by various stress factors in your lifestyle, home or work environment, financial circumstances, personal relationships, and especially any recent experience of trauma or grief. These can take hold of you in an emotionally devastating, debilitating way.

Although there is no way to definitively predict or prevent

Reclaim the Joy of Motherhood

Postpartum Depression, some women may be more likely to get it than others. One of the strongest predictors that a woman might get Postpartum Depression is depression or anxiety during pregnancy, especially in the third trimester.[11] Some other risk factors might be:

- Prior or family history of depression or anxiety

- Difficulties with your spouse or partner

- Stressful life events, such as losing a job, moving, or the death or illness of a loved one

- Financial distress

- Lack of social support or adequate help with childcare

- Caring for a child with behavioral or temperamental challenges

- Low self-esteem

- Being a single mom, or under the age of twenty

- Unplanned or unwanted pregnancy

- Difficult or traumatic birth experience

- Alcohol, drug, or tobacco abuse

- A sick or colicky baby

These risk factors do not automatically cause Postpartum Depression. You might never experience PPD, despite having many of the above factors present in your daily life. Or you might get PPD with only one risk factor, or sometimes even none.

It is important to remember that each woman is different and should not be subject to comparison with others.

Do you have any risk factors that may be contributing to what's going on with you? What is going on in your life to cause you stress? Use this space to explain:

_____

_____

_____

_____

_____

_____

_____

There is never a need to feel ashamed, guilty, or embarrassed about being diagnosed with or having Postpartum Depression. It is no different than needing medical attention for an infection or other illness. Though it is not often openly talked about, unfortunately sometimes even between medical professionals, it is real. You are not crazy for feeling the way you do. You are not imagining things. You are not a bad mother.

I am so happy to tell you that Postpartum Depression will not last forever. With the proper care and treatment you will beat this, and reclaim the joy of motherhood!

SECTION II

It's Not My Fault

CHAPTER SIX

The Battle of "What If?"

"There are no shortcuts to any place worth going."

- Beverly Sills

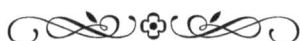

After the night of my terrifying chest pains, and the morning when I discovered that PPD was real, I sank even deeper into the darkness. Over the next few days, I hit rock bottom.

Time seemed to jump around inconsistently from moment to moment, every second overflowing with sadness, listlessness, and guilt. Nothing penetrated me except the thoughts that pierced my heart. I was hunkered down into the barracks of battle, in protect and survive mode.

My body was going through the motions, taking care of the things that absolutely had to get done: nursing Brayden, putting him to sleep, figuring out food for Zack, Will, and, barely, for myself. I knew I had to do these things, so I did them. I knew, because I was feeding Brayden, that I needed to drink water and eat food. So I would drink a little water and eat maybe a fruit cup or some crackers and cheese. Beyond that, I just tried to zone out as much as I could. I probably spent most of my time lying on the couch and watching TV. It is difficult now to remember how that time actually passed; outwardly, I was doing almost nothing, but inside my mind, a war was raging that threatened to tear me apart.

I don't know if the phone rang at all, but I wouldn't have answered it. I didn't want to talk to anybody. No one could talk to me, no one could do or say anything to pierce the shield I had constructed around myself. And this shield I had built for protection had become a prison. Inside the walls, it was much, much more dangerous than in the outside world. Inside my mind, the battle for survival was consuming me, using up all my resources and leaving me battered, bruised, and completely exhausted.

By this time, Will and I were almost not talking at all. It was like living with a roommate. He would go to work, pick up Zackery on his way home, and then pretty much leave me alone. He really didn't know how to deal with me. He had tried so many times to reach out, in so many ways, and every time I had shut him down. I was shut down, myself. I was almost beyond help.

Sometimes, while Will was at work and Zackery was at daycare—when it was just me and Brayden in the house—crazy thoughts would pop into my mind as if they belonged and deserved to be there. What if I just got in the car, right now, and drove away? What if I left Brayden all alone in the house? What if I just…left? I didn't know where I would go; I hadn't planned anything out. I just thought about getting in the car and driving far, far away. I had thoughts about never coming back. What would Will do? Would Zackery remember me? Brayden would be too young. Would I leave forever, or just for a little while? Would I tell anyone where I was going?

These thoughts, a terrifying stream of what-ifs, had started plaguing me day in and day out. They were like arrows flying from an unseen bow, piercing my heart and my head over and over, deeper and deeper. I didn't want those thoughts. Where did they come from? They couldn't have been from me; they didn't make any sense. But no matter how hard I tried to stop them, they only got worse.

I dreaded every time Brayden would cry in hunger, because breastfeeding him was still painful due to his problematic latch. I knew the pain that I would have to endure, just to feed him the milk we both so very much wanted him to have. What if I just didn't feed my baby? my brain would ask. What if I just let him cry, hungry, starving, helpless? Could I actually do that? Would I actually do that?

The thoughts kept getting worse, darker, more violent and frightening.

What if I drove off a cliff, Thelma and Louise style?

What would happen if I just closed my eyes, with the boys in the backseat?

What if I put Brayden in the dryer?

What if I took a baseball bat to Zackery?

What would happen?

Reclaim the Joy of Motherhood

The thoughts were so incredibly evil. The unwanted, awful idea of torturing my own children tortured me. I couldn't tell anybody about this. If I so much as hinted at what I was thinking, any sane person would call Child Protective Services and get my kids taken away from me. I would be arrested and thrown in jail, Will would have to be a single dad, and I would die of guilt, far, far away from the family I loved.

I would never succumb to these thoughts—how could I? Or maybe that's what I was so afraid of. What if these ideas somehow made their way deep into my brain, to the part of me that believed it necessary to take action upon them? What if I couldn't get rid of them? What if I followed through on one of those crazy, demented cognitions?

What if?

You hear stories on the news, every so often, about a mother killing her children. There was one who drove her car into a lake or pond, with her children strapped into their car seats. Then there was the baby who would not stop crying and crying and crying and crying and crying, until ultimately the caregiver shook the baby so hard that the baby died. You watch those things on the news and your heart sinks. How in the world could someone do such a thing to such a tiny, innocent being? How is it possible? What could possibly have been going through their deranged mind?

In some bizarre way—which angered and disgusted and frightened me—I understood how they could have gone so far as to believe that hurting a child was their answer. The war in their mind must have been raging too...and they lost!

I didn't want to lose. I was trapped in a terrifying battle of split-second decisions, and losing a battle meant I could lose the war.

It's terrifying to think that you might let a torturous thought or a vicious voice in, and not have the power, the strength, or the control to overcome it—losing control of what you know is right and wrong, good and bad, helpful and punishable. Faltering for a mere split second decision could seal your fate in guilt without forgiveness, forever.

I was afraid of getting to that point. To me, that's what depression meant: voices and thoughts and actions I wouldn't be able to control. I had always been in control of my life. Hearing stories about mothers going crazy and murdering their children, their husbands, and themselves—I did not want to be one of them. But now, under constant siege from the most frightening enemy I had ever faced, I feared I was losing control.

Part of me knew what I had to do: I needed to get help. But the guilt I was experiencing was enormous. I felt so guilty that Will had to help me with every little task; guilty that my friends and family were already helping so much; but mostly, I felt guilty that I had let this happen to myself. I couldn't face the shame of admitting that I had this disease, this illness that made me officially weak. How could I have let this happen? How could I burden my friends and Will by asking for more help?

Reclaim the Joy of Motherhood

And what would people say about me if I admitted that something might be wrong? Everyone knew me as a smart, happy, positive, out-going, driven, determined woman. Conceding to PPD would mean that everyone's image of me would be washed away by the image of depression, weakness, and gloom. It meant I would no longer be able to lie and hide behind fake smiles and say, "I'm great, motherhood is wonderful!" It meant I would have to be honest with what was really going on.

The prospect of admitting that I was in trouble was nearly as terrifying as the idea of what would happen if I didn't get help. All I could do was hide, paralyzed, while my mind raced in circles and the battle for my sanity raged on. I felt so alone and overwhelmed.

Of course, even there at rock bottom, hiding broken and bruised inside my fortress, I was not truly alone. I was surrounded by people who loved me: Will, Zackery and Brayden, Elisa and Courtney, Marlena, my father and sister. They all cared about me, but there at my lowest point there was only one person who could get through to me, the one who had never left my side because he actually couldn't: my angel baby, Brayden.

My boys were both so perfect and I loved them both deeply, but behind my impenetrable wall I was as disconnected from them as I could be. Zackery, poor Zackery. What he must have been feeling or thinking of his disengaged mother. Thank goodness he was young. I hope he won't remember the dark anguish I was in.

Brayden, though, would not let me fade away. He saw me. When he would just look at me with those innocent little eyes and smile, I could see that he still wanted me, still loved me, still needed me. And he was still utterly dependent on me for everything. He was the one thing that I could not disappear from, because without me, he would die. No one else could feed him, or hold him like I did while we slept. Without me to take care of him, his life would be over. Yes, Will needed me and Zackery needed me, but Brayden NEEDED me.

Still, need was not the message Brayden was sending me, not at all. With his clear eyes and his beautiful smile, he was telling me to remember what is important: to be present in the moment, to put aside my worries and focus on living. He was telling me that I was loved, and that things were okay. His love cut right through the battle in my mind, past all the confusion and bedlam, and he was simply there. The evil thoughts and darkness could not stop him. My mental war didn't matter; all that mattered was love.

With his pure, innocent love, and with no idea what he was doing or how he was affecting me, my baby Brayden saved my life.

CHAPTER SEVEN

Asking For Help

"You gain strength, courage and confidence by every experience in which you really stop to look fear in the face. You are able to say to yourself, 'I have lived through this horror. I can take the next thing that comes along.' You must do the thing you think you cannot do."

- Eleanor Roosevelt

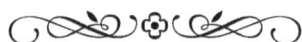

After two or three days at rock bottom, there was nowhere to go but up and out of the deep dark hole. I could no longer deny that I needed to talk to someone, but whom? There was just one person with whom I might be able to talk openly: someone who just might understand, without needing to hear every evil detail of the demons I was fighting in the devil's playground. This person was my doula, Marlena. She was the one person who could pull a half-forgotten smile out of the graveyard of my heart, who could convince me to take just one little step toward a new life.

I don't even remember dialing, but I found myself on the phone with her. "Something's not right," I said in a trembling voice. "I'm scared."

Marlena immediately told me to come to her house. It seemed like an incredibly hard thing to do, but she coaxed me into it. "Come over. We should talk in person." Somehow, through the deep fog muffling my mind, I found a way to get Brayden and myself there.

I can't remember the details of what happened next. The words we spoke and the emotions battling for my heart—it is all drowned in that fog. But I remember the scene at Marlena's home so clearly and crisply, a vivid picture. I had placed a patterned receiving blanket on the floor next to Brayden's gray and red infant carrier. It was light blue with dark blue stars, to match the soft, light blue onesie and pants he was wearing. I sat on the dark green couch. The walls were adorned with beautifully patterned wallpaper. My doula's house shone with love. Warm, smiling family pictures surrounded me throughout the room, unafraid of the cold chill inside my heart.

Brayden, as usual, kept his eyes on his mother—always following me. He was happily smiling, waving and kicking his arms and legs with delight and joy, just like he was supposed to. I agonized over my internal pain and not being able to express the same delight and joy as he did. Brayden was the happiest, most beautiful, perfect little angel boy. Why, oh why, was I not happy?

I don't remember the exact words we exchanged, but I remember being there for several hours, talking mostly, crying the entire time. My floodgates opened. I confided my terrifying thoughts that wouldn't go away; how I was scared that my brain would mistake a thought of harming myself or my family as a good idea that I would then act upon, leaving me a statistic like one of those women you hear about on the evening news. I told Marlena that all I wanted to do was love and feed my baby, but that I dreaded every time Brayden cried because I knew the pain it would cause me to nurse him. I shared how very tired I was, exhausted, fatigued beyond relief, yet I couldn't ever sleep. I told her about the physical pain in my chest from several nights before: the constant backache, muscle aches, and headaches; how I lacked the desire to do anything at all; how I didn't want to get dressed, brush my teeth, or take a shower because it was too much effort and "what's the point?"

I told Marlena that I just wanted to shut everyone out. I didn't want to talk to anyone about anything. I didn't want to call anybody back, even my best friend, Elisa. I didn't want to talk to Will about how my day was going because I didn't know how my day was going, other than it being foggy, unclear, and unfocused. I couldn't remember anything anymore—which was completely opposite of the person I used to be. I didn't want to go outside and take a walk or go for a hike—all things that I used to love doing, alone and with Will or Zackery, even before Brayden came along. I felt so guilty for feeling helpless and sad all the time. I told Marlena that I just felt numb, and couldn't ever stop crying.

Miraculously, she understood my numbness, and why I was so torn and crippled with guilt. She understood my not being able to express happiness over the bundle of joy that innocently depended on me for everything. My doula understood. She said she already knew what was wrong with me, but hadn't told me earlier because I wasn't ready to hear it. She knew. She knew everything about what I was going through. Not one single moment or thought I described to her was shocking or shameful. She told me that this wasn't anything I could have prevented or controlled on my own. She knew what it was, and what I had to do.

Marlena made me promise to call my doctor immediately, tell him I had Postpartum Depression, and ask for help. She didn't want to frighten me, but she did want to make me see just how serious Postpartum Depression was. She stressed that if I didn't ask for help, she didn't know what might happen to me, Brayden, or even Zackery for that matter.

The last hours at Marlena's house were like a dream as the fog closed in again. When it was time for me to leave, the thought of being on my own again scared me. I knew I would be going home to an empty house, just me and Brayden. Marlena repeated the same instructions over and over to me. She wanted me to hear and remember them, because she could see I was trying so hard not to believe her. "Go right home. Call your doctor," she said, pronouncing every word slowly and clearly, making sure I understood. "Tell him you have Postpartum Depression—not that you think you have it, but that you have it." She wouldn't let me leave until I promised I would make the phone call. Then she lightened the burden a bit by offering me hope. She reminded me that I would be okay. Postpartum

Depression wasn't permanent. I hadn't done anything wrong. It was an illness, and it could be treated.

My whole world had become a clouded mystery that made no sense. It wasn't anything at all like I had expected my life would be. It certainly wasn't the beautiful, peaceful, happy vision I had imagined. It was cold and dark, so very, very dark, with barely the flicker of a dying candle left in the distance. My world was lonely, and I didn't believe that there was anyone who could break through the iron gates or welded shackles that bound me there. But Marlena knew. One of the most important things she said to me was that I had her to lean on—that I could count on her. Not only did she understand where I was, she knew how to get me out.

It wasn't a long drive home, but to me it felt like an eternity. I cried all the way to our driveway. I cried because I was scared. I cried because I was sad. I cried because I was afraid for me, for Brayden, for Zackery, and for Will. I cried because someone really cared. I cried because there was now someone reaching in through the iron gates and trying to rescue me.

I walked into my empty house, went directly to my room and placed Brayden on the floor. He was still asleep in his carrier from the car ride home. I knew what I had to do: I had to call my doctor. But I couldn't. I stared at the phone and it glared back at me, taunting me to pick it up. I couldn't do it! I was petrified of what my doctor would say. I was terrorized by the words I would hear myself say to him: "I have Postpartum Depression."

Reclaim the Joy of Motherhood

I have always been a strong woman, a woman of my word. I had made a promise to my doula that I would call. I took the deepest breath I knew how to take in at that moment. I reached out and gripped the cold, smooth, silver phone and put it to my ear. But somehow, even though I knew the doctor's number by heart, it was not the number I dialed. I knew I needed to be in a place of immense courage in order to ask for help, and I just wasn't there yet. All I could do was cry, gasping for breath between each heavy tear that streamed down my face.

The phone was ringing on the other end. I was so conflicted. I prayed that no one would answer, and begged that someone would.

"Hello?" said a familiar voice.

"Hi," I barely whispered in response.

Courtney was my close friend. She had a little girl about two months older than Brayden, and we had a lot in common, including sharing the same doula. We often spent time together on playdates or just having coffee, sometimes as a group with Marlena. I trusted Courtney. I sought her understanding and compassion. But what would she think of me?

With a quivering voice, I began to confide my dark secret to Courtney. "Something is wrong with me. I'm not myself." I awkwardly shared the events of the past seventy-two hours with her. I revealed to her the anxiety pain in my chest, the negative voices in my head, my fears and fatigue. I told her how alone and helpless I felt, bound to this hell I was in. I had lost all hope and joy.

To my surprise, she already knew. She and our doula had already talked. There were more people trying to break into my prison than I had realized.

I was committed to keeping the promise I had made to Marlena, but I needed more help. "Tell me exactly, word for word, what I am supposed to say when I call my doctor," I pleaded. Courtney repeated the same thing my doula had told me to say: "I have Postpartum Depression. I don't think I have it, I have it."

"You can do this, Pam," she encouraged. "You have to do this."

And then she was gone. Once again, it was just me and the phone. Fear paralyzed me. My heart began to beat faster, my eyes swelled with tears, and I couldn't see. My palms were sweaty, and my hands were shaking. There was no one else in the house except little sleeping Brayden. He could not make the call for me. I began begging myself to call. This was the hardest thing I could imagine doing, but I slowly gathered enough courage to pick up the phone. This time I dialed my doctor. I knew his number well; I had dialed it so many times before, but those were on happy occasions. This time, I dialed as if it were my last hope to be rescued from the devil's snare.

The receptionist answered. "This is Pamela Zimmer. I have Postpartum Depression, I don't think I have it. I have it. I need help." I'm lucky that she was able to understand what I was saying through my tears. The desperation in my voice must have made her realize how serious this was, and that scheduling an appointment in the morning was not going to be an option.

"Stay on the phone," she said. "Don't hang up. I am going to get the doctor to come talk with you right now."

I felt so blessed that I would be able to speak to him over the phone right away, and not have to wait until a morning office visit. I don't know what would have happened if I had endured another night of the frightful unknown, all alone with the knowledge that I had PPD. I didn't want to have one more night of guilt—guilt for getting PPD; for not telling anyone; for not pulling my weight as Brayden and Zackery's mother; and for being tired, fatigued, exhausted, and indecisive, all along with all of the other symptoms of PPD.

My doctor's voice finally came through the phone. He assured me that everything would be all right. Together, we agreed that I would try antidepressant medication. He called in the prescription; I just had to pick it up.

Now, how in the world was I going to manage doing that?

Everything felt like such a blur. After everything that had happened, even the smallest task felt impossible. Brayden was going to wake up any minute, and I would need to nurse him— that was the only thing I knew for sure. Time seemed to move in slow motion. I could only function moment by moment. I couldn't think, I couldn't feel, I couldn't focus on anything if it wasn't in that moment. Brayden was here in this moment, so I cared for him. Other than that, I was numb.

My day felt surreal. *What had just happened? What had I done today? What was going on? This couldn't be my life. This was not me!*

I decided to make one more call—to my husband. With a trembling, vacant calmness, I dialed his phone and asked him if he would please go pick up a prescription for me on the way home.

"Prescription? For what?" he asked. "Anti-depressants," I answered matter-of-factly, trying to hold back the tears. "I have Postpartum Depression."

There was a short pause, and then he asked me why I hadn't talked to him about it sooner. I was embarrassed, ashamed, scared, and detached; all I could tell him was that I didn't know. The conversation didn't include much more. I didn't know how to tell him or how to talk about what I had been feeling. The reality was that I hadn't been feeling anything at all. I was mentally and emotionally blank.

Will left work early that day to pick up the two things he knew I couldn't: pills and our son, Zackery. I did the only thing I was good at doing lately. I cried.

CHAPTER EIGHT

When This Is You

"There are wounds that never show on the body that are deeper and more hurtful than anything that bleeds."

- Laurell K. Hamilton

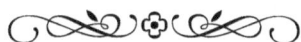

By now, you may be feeling that something is going on with you, or you may be completely sure that something is wrong, or you may be thinking that your situation isn't as bad as mine was. I have shared my story with you as a way of throwing out a lifeline, a thread of hope that can carry you to safety if you are truly lost. But the truth is that everyone's experience is different. Now it is time for you to begin documenting your own story. In this chapter, I will ask you some questions, and give you a place to write freely about what is happening in your heart and in your head.

There are many different symptoms of Postpartum Depression, and since each person is different, it is very important not to compare yourself to others. It is also important to understand that you might not have any of the most common symptoms, or that you might experience them all in varying degrees. Whatever your circumstance, whatever your scenario, whatever you are feeling: listen to your body and your heart. You don't need to be ashamed or embarrassed, or try to hide what is really going on. You are a beautiful, unique, amazing individual and you need to be heard.

And what if you don't know for sure what is happening to you? What do you do when you feel in your heart that something is not quite right? Whom do you call? How do you know if what you are experiencing is full-blown Postpartum Depression, or just the Baby Blues? What does it mean?

When you notice a difference in yourself—whether it is all the time, or only during certain moments—from feeling withdrawn, sad, or guilty, to not wanting to care for yourself or your baby: the first thing you should do is write it down. Write down the time of day the feeling came over you, what you were doing, what your baby was doing, anything that seems relevant. Get a journal, or even just a dedicated piece of paper, to keep track. You can even use this book to take notes in. Write down each different feeling or symptom. Take note of how long you feel that way, and whether it is something that comes and goes. This might sound daunting, especially with everything else you are likely going through, but it is an essential step.

I never wrote down what I was feeling until after I was diagnosed, and I wish I had. It might have made it easier to get help sooner if I had been more aware of my physical and emotional patterns and symptoms. On the other hand, I also wasn't fully aware that I was feeling anything, other than the fatigue that I thought was normal. If I had seen the words on the page, the reality of my situation might have become clear much sooner.

Because I wasn't aware of my body, my emotions, my mind, I could not move forward. Awareness, therefore, was the very first step in my journey of healing, and it should be a part of yours, too. No matter what you are feeling—whether you have full-blown PPD or just the Baby Blues, or are just having a terrible month—becoming more aware of your reality can only help by showing you the opportunities to begin healing.

I cannot give you the answer to finding your own awareness, but I can share with you what works for me. When I am quiet, when I pause and just focus on my breath, that is when the awareness of my body, mind, and spirit presents itself. It takes practice, and it takes patience. When I began working on improving my self-awareness, it was difficult. I had to remove myself from all external noise and distractions. I needed to sit by myself in a peaceful, quiet place, often closing my eyes to maintain focus. I had to concentrate on breathing in and breathing out, breathing in and breathing out. It has taken me many years to get to where I am now, to a point where I am completely aware of my body, my thoughts, and my heart. You will get there too. In the beginning, though, just try to be quiet and still, and listen to your body. It will not take long for your awareness to increase.

With improved focus and awareness, you are able to observe and document anything and everything that seems abnormal or at odds with your true self. There is no right or wrong way to do this; there is no symptom or emotion or feeling that is too big or too little to make note of. There is only you, trusting in your heart.

Along with awareness comes asking for help. If you are anything like me, you will feel scared, embarrassed, ashamed, and uneasy. You might also feel denial, or that you don't need help. You might think, "Oh, this will pass. It's just a little mood swing because I'm so tired. If I can just get some sleep I'll feel better." This is what I felt for months, until I was ready to accept I had Postpartum Depression. In your case, I hope it will pass; but if it does not go away, you will have your journal to look back on.

For many women, before you can talk to somebody else about what is happening, you have to know what it is you want to talk to them about. You need to be able to understand and process what is happening with you. Now is your time to let it all out. Be aware and honest, and just start writing it down.

Questions For You

How are you feeling?

_____

_____

What did you do today?

_____

_____

Did you cry today?

_____

Is anything making you worried or anxious? What is it?

_____

_____

Are you feeling guilty? What about?

_____

_____

When was the last time you slept well?

_____

_____

How many hours are you sleeping?

_____

_____

How often are you getting out of the house?

_____

_____

How often are you getting alone time, without your baby? How does it make you feel?

_____

_____

When was the last time you called a friend?

_____

_____

When was the last time somebody called you? Did you answer?

_____

_____

**When was the last time you gave someone a hug, or said
"I love you"?**

_____

_____

When was the last time you made a decision?

_____

_____

Did you eat today? Did you drink any water?

_____

_____

Did you take a shower? Brush your teeth? Change your clothes?

_____

_____

What else is going on?

_____

_____

_____

_____

_____

_____

Some of your answers already may be giving you a wake-up call. If they are, listen!

When you experience the symptoms of Postpartum Depression, do not be afraid. Do not ignore and cast aside your feelings. Trust your gut, trust your instinct, trust your women's intuition. This is real, it is happening, but you are not alone. There is help out there; all you have to do is speak up. Believe that someone will be there to listen. If I can do it, so can you, and together we can help each other.

CHAPTER NINE

Fact or Fiction?

"We must not allow other people's limited perceptions to define us."

- Virginia Satir

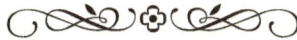

When I started my research into Postpartum Depression, so many things that had never made sense suddenly became crystal clear. PPD made it real: Everything that had been going on with me had a cause that was based in my body's chemistry. I wasn't imagining it, and I hadn't done anything terrible to deserve it. The more I read and researched, the more it all made sense. Once again in my life, I was discovering how true it is that "you don't know what you don't know." There was so much I never knew about what was happening inside my own skin!

One of the biggest hurdles that women with PPD must overcome is the huge lack of information and education around this very common illness. I remember when I talked to Elisa on the phone before my diagnosis, and her reaction to my complaints was to tell me to "mommy up." That made me feel so hurt and frustrated. I couldn't just mommy up! She didn't understand what I was going through, not at all. That ended up being part of the reason why I didn't talk to anybody about what was going on with me: I really felt that they would not understand. Now I know that I didn't understand either, and that none of us really knew enough about what might be happening to me. When you can't share what is going on with you in a way that other people can understand, it all feels pointless. Why bother trying?

When you're pregnant, and right after you give birth, you might have access to some information about PPD, or at least about the Baby Blues. I remember reading somewhere, long back before I had Zackery, that it was normal to feel down for a while, even to cry. But then it would go away, the joy of motherhood would take over, and your life would become wonderful again! For so many women, this is a false message. The reality is that sometimes it gets worse.

I've mentioned before that my dad was the first person to tell me that it was okay to cry. Later, I came to realize that he had seen my mother fight her own battle with depression. When I was nine or ten years old, my mom was diagnosed with depression and admitted into an in-patient facility near our home. I don't remember much about her diagnosis or what happened to trigger it, other than her being sad all the time. My dad took my sister and I to visit her quite often, and she only stayed in the facility for about a month. I remember visiting her one day, and she was doing an arts-and-craft project: a ceramic apple that she had painted in rainbow stripes to match the logo design for Apple Computer (the company where my dad worked at the time).

I believe Dad still has that apple. I remember that moment because she smiled and seemed happy. There was a light, a shift, a hope in her that she hadn't shown or probably even experienced herself for a long, long time.

Before that moment, my mom was sad. When she cried, she tried to hide her tears as much as she could (much like I did), but we all saw them at times. I didn't talk to my parents much about what was going on. I didn't know what to say; I was young. Ultimately, it was a secret that my mother held in her own heart, tightly locked away.

I have no idea whether my mother might have struggled with PPD, after suffering two miscarriages of her own. I know that, when she was pregnant with me, she was so scared of miscarrying again that she would not even let anybody take a photo of her. I don't know what was really happening in my mom's heart. As emotionally driven as she was, I know it must have been devastating for her to lose two children in that way, but she kept her pain private and secret. Even later, when she was undergoing chemotherapy for her leukemia, she never shared with us the pain and anguish she felt. After she passed away, my dad found letters and journals detailing her true feelings. It was heartbreaking to think that she was not able to tell anyone about the pain and loneliness she experienced while fighting through something like that.

Later, when I was going through my own darkness, I think part of me reacted like my mother would have. I kept my pain a secret. I didn't want to burden anyone with it, and I didn't want to be perceived as weak. I also didn't want to be locked away in a facility for sad, depressed, broken people. I didn't want Will to have to bring Zackery and Brayden to visit their mother in some strange, unknown place that wasn't home, like my dad had to do with my sister and I. I didn't want to have those negative things associated with me. I didn't want that stigma.

Having to admit that I had PPD meant, at first, that I was flawed, broken, damaged. It meant I wasn't the strong, in-control woman I thought I was. It meant there was something wrong with me, something I should have prevented. It meant that it was my fault, that there was something more I could have done but didn't. This is what I thought, before I really knew what PPD was. This is what so many women still believe. This is completely untrue.

As I learned more about the facts of PPD, all those fictions began to vanish, chased away by the truth. Even in the first few days, as it began to sink in that my illness was something real, I started to see the signs all around me. After starting my own research, I made a post on my Facebook wall:

"Postpartum Depression is nothing to be ashamed of, and it doesn't mean you are a bad mother."

Almost right away, two different women told me that they had gone through it themselves. Each of them had children that were a few years old! All that time, I had never seen the slightest indication of what they had been going through. Still, to this day, I hear from old friends and acquaintances, even strangers, who share their stories with me. So many of the women in my extended circles—even in my own family—have fought depression at various stages of their lives, and many of them after having a child. But absolutely nobody talks about it. It's like a dirty little secret.

It makes me furious that women feel they have to hide depression. It's not like they have done anything to deserve it! Over the generations, we have developed this myth that you just need to shut up and swallow your pain—that weakness is a fault, not a reality that we all share.

For me, talking openly about my PPD was incredibly powerful. Once I started being honest and unashamed, it was like the floodgates opened and I was surrounded with love and support. One of the biggest changes was in my relationship with Elisa. The more I learned and shared with her, the more she was able to see and understand the reality that I had been living. Once she understood, she was completely empathetic, and she has been there for me through every step of my recovery. What a change truth and openness can bring! As soon as I stopped hiding the pain inside myself, as soon as I brought it out into the light where my best friend could see it, she was able to be a true friend to me in the way she always meant to be.

This is why my mission is to help share the truth about PPD, to shine light on an illness that is kept in darkness. Why should it be? There is no reason for this to be a secret. It is not something to be ashamed of.

So, let's focus on the facts and let the truth dispel the myths. Here is a quiz to test your knowledge of PPD. The answers might surprise you (they certainly surprised me!)

Postpartum Depression: Fact or Fiction?

1. Up to one in five women will experience Postpartum Depression each year.

○ Fact OR ○ Fiction

2. Postpartum Depression is more common than preterm labor.

○ Fact OR ○ Fiction

3. Most women who experience depression receive treatment.

○ Fact OR ○ Fiction

4. Suicide is the third most common cause of mortality in postpartum women.

○ Fact OR ○ Fiction

5. Postpartum Depression affects women within the first few weeks after childbirth.

○ Fact OR ○ Fiction

6. A mother's Postpartum Depression can affect her baby's health and development.

○ Fact OR ○ Fiction

7. Postpartum Depression makes you a bad mother.

○ Fact OR ○ Fiction

8. All women are at risk for Postpartum Depression, regardless of the pregnancy's outcome.

◯ Fact OR ◯ Fiction

9. It is possible to identify risk factors for PPD, even before pregnancy or childbirth.

◯ Fact OR ◯ Fiction

10. Nearly 1,000,000 women suffer from Postpartum Depression each year.

◯ Fact OR ◯ Fiction

11. Postpartum Depression is a disease that can be treated.

◯ Fact OR ◯ Fiction

12. If you have thoughts of harming your baby, you need to be separated from your child(ren) immediately to keep them out of danger.

◯ Fact OR ◯ Fiction

13. Your doctor will tell you if you might have Postpartum Depression.

◯ Fact OR ◯ Fiction

1. FACT. An estimated nine to sixteen percent of mothers are diagnosed with Postpartum Depression each year (which in itself is a pretty big number, with a pretty big range). This estimate does not take into account all the unreported cases of women with PPD, so in reality, the percentage may be as high as twenty percent, or one in five.

2. FACT. Postpartum Depression is the most common complication associated with childbirth and pregnancy. It occurs more often than preterm labor (twelve percent of women), pre-eclampsia (five to eight percent), low birth weight (eight percent), ectopic pregnancy (two percent), and gestational diabetes (four to seven percent). All women receiving proper prenatal care are screened for gestational diabetes during their pregnancy, but most women are not screened for depression. Perhaps this is because there is no blood test or definitive screening method.

3. FICTION. Only half of pregnant women who experience depression receive treatment. Fifty-four percent of non-pregnant women (either from a successful birth or a miscarriage) who experience depression receive treatment. Up to twenty-six percent of all women with untreated depression say they have not sought treatment because of the negative stigma. Forty-two percent are opposed to treatment.

4. FICTION. In truth, suicide is the second most common cause of mortality in postpartum women, accounting for approximately twenty percent of postpartum deaths. A shockingly high number, I know! Furthermore, out of the women who are diagnosed with Postpartum Depression, one in five (twenty percent) experience thoughts of harming themselves.

5. FICTION. Up to eighty percent of all women who have just given birth experience the Baby Blues, which last anywhere from two to six weeks. Baby Blues are very common, and usually do not require medical treatment. When the Baby Blues don't go away, it is time to consider Postpartum Depression, which can set in any time from a month to a year or more after childbirth.

6. FACT. Studies of mothers diagnosed with PPD show an increased number of sick infants, with some leading to emergency visits and others hospitalization. In addition, children of mothers with Postpartum Depression are more likely to have difficulties with sleep and eating, have more frequent temper tantrums and hyperactivity, and exhibit other behavioral challenges. They are also more likely to experience delays in cognitive, emotional, and social development, potentially leading to an early onset of depression themselves. This is not to say that every one of the 400,000 children born to depressed mothers each year will show these signs; it just means the risk and the potential is greater.

7. FICTION. Kristin Hodson, founder of The Healing Group, says she meets many mothers who believe they are caught in an either/or situation: "Either I'm a good mom (and good moms don't have PPD), or I'm a bad mom because I have PPD." That is simply not the case, Hodson says. "Moms can be good moms and experience PPD, and they deserve to get help and get better. They are not how they are feeling. What they are experiencing are symptoms of PPD, and those are treatable."

"Many women experiencing the symptoms of a postpartum mood disorder are frightened to disclose their symptoms," says Valerie McManus, a social worker and psychologist. "They fear they will be labeled as a bad mother or misinterpreted as not valuing the blessing that is their child. One of the most powerful stigmas associated with postpartum mood disorders is that women who suffer from PPD are at substantial risk for harming their children. In fact, Postpartum Depression is simply one variation fitting under the umbrella term of postpartum mood disorder."

8. FACT. Postpartum Depression does not discriminate. It does not matter how old you are, what your social or economic status is, what nationality you are, or where you live. It also doesn't matter if you had a successful live birth. Postpartum Depression affects women who have suffered a miscarriage or a stillbirth, who have adopted children, and it even affects ten to fourteen percent of new fathers. There is a myth that Postpartum Depression occurs only because of the rapid change in hormones after a mother gives birth. This is just one of the factors. Others may include environmental stresses and traumas, financial burden and stress, lack of support and help with the new baby, young maternal age, or a combination of several factors. The key is to understand that Postpartum Depression is not just a simple hormone imbalance.

9. FACT. Research has identified several risk factors that can contribute to PPD. This does NOT mean that every woman with those risk factors will in fact experience it, and it's also possible that you might have PPD without any of the risk factors being present. Nonetheless, being more aware of the risks before a woman even becomes a mother could help her prepare and react sooner if she begins to feel that something is wrong.

"There appears to be a strong correlation between a history of depression or / and anxiety and the development of a postpartum mood disorder," says Valerie McManus. "Further, women who are experiencing high levels of relationship or financial stress also appear at greater risk … While these factors unfortunately seem to contribute to the incidence of postpartum disorders, our ability to correlate them allows for the possibility of pre-screening, preventative safeguards to be put in place, as well as early intervention."

"Signs of PPD often start showing up during pregnancy and really become exacerbated postpartum," says Kristin Hodson. It is theoretically possible for your doctor to screen you for PPD risk while you are still pregnant; however, this is not a common practice in the slightest. Most women do not find out about PPD unless they are diagnosed with it. This is a shame: early screening and detection could save many women from the serious emotional and physical struggles that PPD creates for mothers and for their children.

10. FACT. The estimated number of live births in the United States in 2012 was 3,952,937. Twenty percent of that is nearly 800,000, and again this was in the United States alone. Add to that the percentage of women who are diagnosed with PPD after enduring a miscarriage or stillbirth, or even more tragically an infant death, and we are nearing 1,000,000, if not more—just in America. That's more women than will get diabetes, suffer a stroke, or be diagnosed with breast cancer.

11. FACT. According to www.dictionary.com, disease is defined as follows:

"a disordered or incorrectly functioning organ, part, structure, or system of the body resulting from the effect of genetic or developmental errors, infection, poisons, nutritional deficiency or imbalance, toxicity, or unfavorable environmental factors; illness; sickness; ailment."

To be diagnosed with Postpartum Depression does not mean you did anything wrong, that you are to blame, or that you should feel guilty. It simply means that your body is not functioning properly. There is no completely accurate method to predict or prevent PPD, but it can be treated successfully. The earlier you begin treatment, the more effective it will be.

12. FICTION. Women such as I who have frightening thoughts of hurting their babies may be suffering from Postpartum Obsessive-Compulsive Disorder or another anxiety disorder—not psychosis. "Women often think this is psychosis because they have 'intrusive thoughts' about harming their baby," wellness consultant Stacey Glaesmann says. "I have had women in a hospital psych ward call me to speak to their doctors because they were diagnosed with psychosis and were facing threats of having their babies taken away. Actually, a woman with PP OCD is least likely to harm their baby because the thoughts horrify them. Women with real Postpartum Psychosis have delusions and hallucinations, which are just part of their reality; they don't realize that anything is wrong."

"While postpartum psychosis is a severe and sometimes dangerous disorder, it is also extremely rare," says Valerie McManus. Psychosis does occur for one woman in one thousand; it is much less common than severe anxiety. "Rarer still are instances when a women suffering from postpartum psychosis actually acts out against her baby. Of the few cases where mothers did harm or kill their children, they were acting out of a state of psychosis...We learn of these cases when the women are splayed across every news channel depicted, not as severely ill, but as monsters." This is an unfair depiction, not only to those women, but to any mother who believes that seeking help might result in having her children taken away.

13. FICTION. Your doctor is one of your greatest allies through the entire process of pregnancy and childbirth, but because of the way treatment is structured in our health system, your doctor might not be able to connect with you during that crucial period—the months after you have your baby.

"Just because someone has 'M.D.' after their name doesn't mean they know much about PPD," Glaesmann says. "Considering that up to 20 percent of new moms develop a postpartum mood disorder, I know that many fall through the cracks because of lack of follow-up. Many PPMD advocacy groups are reaching out to pediatricians to train them to ask the 'right' questions and look for telltale signs, because that's who the woman sees the most following her six-week OB check-up. Many moms do not develop symptoms until two to three months postpartum, and some even later than that (when weaning from breastfeeding, for example)."

103

Your OBGYN will probably see you six weeks after you give birth, at which point it is fairly likely that you could be suffering from the Baby Blues. After that, you might not talk to your doctor again for another nine months or a year. During this period, there is no way your doctor could know if you are suffering. Even if he or she gives you a pamphlet on depression—which not all doctors do—many mothers, myself included, will barely read it because we think it could not happen to us.

"Given that there exist several research-supported risk factors increasing the likelihood of a woman developing a postpartum mood disorder," says McManus, "why are we not routinely assessing each pregnant woman's potential risk? With such information, we would be able to arm them with the resources necessary to potentially reduce symptoms and increase intervention timeframes."

I feel very strongly that health care providers for pregnant women and new moms must be more involved in screening for postpartum disorders. This is a topic that we'll revisit again later in the book; for now, just be aware that while your doctor may be following protocol perfectly, he or she can still miss the signs of PPD. If you think something is wrong, the best thing to do is to speak up.

CHAPTER TEN

Supportive Open Strategies (SOS)

"I've learned that people will forget what you said, people will forget what you did, but people will never forget how you made them feel."

- Maya Angelou

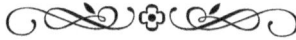

You have been lost at sea for far too long. Set adrift without a map or even an oar to navigate the waters, you've been floating at the whims of the wind and the current. You're exhausted and hopeless, barely surviving. But now, finally, you can see help approaching. It's a ship, and on its decks are all your friends, your family, your doctor, even your baby. They are so close, all you have to do is call out for help, and they can reach down to lift you up.

But what will they think when they see you, bedraggled, sick, exhausted, and barely able to fight the thrashing waves? What if they think you're weak? What if they judge you for getting lost in the first place? What if you are "that lady who got lost at sea" for the rest of your life?

If you really were a castaway and rescue was nearby, of course you would call out for help and never worry about what people thought of you. But depression is never this clear-cut. Your friends might not have noticed anything wrong with you. You might not even be sure of exactly what is happening. You might feel guilty, weak, beyond saving. Above all, you might be so afraid of judgment that you don't even want to ask for help.

It is normal to be afraid, but the danger and judgment you are imagining are not completely real. Your feelings of shame and fear are real, but they are also side effects of depression. Your fear is creating a false vision of reality. As I discovered when I finally asked for help, nobody judged me. Not at all. In fact, when I finally mustered up the courage to say something, I was immediately enveloped in loving support. When I finally made an SOS call, my friends and family were right there to help lift me above the waves.

Now it is time for you to do the same thing. If there is one thing I want you to know, it is that you don't need to be afraid to speak up. You will be surprised at how supportive people actually are, once you begin to ask for their help.

In this chapter, I'm going to share with you some of the ways you can reach out. These are suggestions, based on my own experience. I can't say what your experience will be, but I believe that, as you work through these strategies, you will find solutions that can work for you. By the end of this chapter, I believe that you will be ready to call out an SOS and begin your journey back to the safe, sunny shore.

SOS #1: Sharing With Your Partner

There is one person who probably already knows something is wrong: the person you live with. (For many women, this is your husband or partner; for others, it might be your mother or even a friend. If you don't live with another adult, it's okay to skip to #2.) Not only does your partner see you every day, whether it's a good day or bad; he or she (hopefully) shares household duties with you, and has probably figured out that your chores aren't getting done for the same reason that you're crying a lot and never taking a shower. Something is wrong, and the person you share a home with is the most likely to already know.

That doesn't mean that talking to your partner will be easy. I actually did not talk to Will about my depression at first. I didn't tell him about my 3am chest pains. I didn't share with him the information I had found about Postpartum Depression, or that the symptoms matched mine. I did not even talk to him about my diagnosis. I simply asked him to pick up the medication for me— but that was the first step in asking for Will's help. And the truth is that he had already been supporting me every step of the way.

Will was my rock, and without him I don't know what I would have done. He did almost everything for me when I wasn't able to do it myself. Even after my diagnosis, he continued to take care of everything he could—even while studying for his exams and going to work every day. And every day he would ask me the same question: "How are you doing?" At first, my answer was always the same, too: "Fine," or "Okay." But over time, I started to open up about what was going on with me.

I was afraid to talk to Will because I didn't want to burden him more. He was already carrying so much weight for our family. But as I opened up, I learned that talking to Will about my feelings was not adding to his burden, but actually helping us rebuild our relationship. When I stopped shutting him out, we were able to connect again, and things got easier for both of us. Your own situation at home might be vastly different from mine, of course, but if you feel safe talking about your feelings with your partner, you might find that he or she already knows, loves you unconditionally, and may even welcome your decision to start seeking help.

SOS #2: Asking a Friend Or Mentor For Help

When I was finally ready to make my own SOS call, the first person I called was my doula; the second person was a close friend. These two women not only told me that I needed to talk to a doctor, but they actually gave me the precise words to say to him. Then they made me promise to make the phone call, and would not take "no" for an answer.

When you are hopelessly drifting without an anchor, you need someone who is strong enough to set you on the right course and give you a push. For you, that might be your best friend, or it might be a therapist. It could be a trusted spiritual advisor, or a mentor who has been through what you are experiencing. What matters is that it is someone you can trust completely, because you know they want the best for you. You can put your fate in this person's hands, and know that they will guide you toward safety and healing.

I hope you have such a friend or counselor in your own life. If you do not feel that there is somebody to guide you through the next step, I hope you will reach out to me, and let me be this person for you. I have been where you are, and I can help you find the words and the strength to say them out loud, because I have done it myself. I will not steer you wrong.

SOS #3: Talking To Your Doctor

At a certain point, you will need to speak with a healthcare professional—ideally, your OBGYN or primary physician. Like me, you may not be brave or clear enough to do this right away. It is totally fine to talk to the people you trust most at first. However, PPD is an illness that, left untreated, can do permanent damage to your life and your family. I hope that this will never happen to you. Just to be safe, please, call a doctor as soon as you are able.

For me, this was the most difficult step. I was nearly paralyzed by my fear—fear that I was making it up, fear that I was not making it up, fear that talking to a doctor would make it real, fear that I would be sent to a facility, fear that I would be ignored, fear that I would be judged. It was overwhelming. Thank goodness I had my friends to put the words in my mouth. You may be feeling the same, but do not let the fear take over. Be patient with yourself, and be brave. This is the hardest, scariest part of the entire process: admitting that you are lost, and asking for help. No matter how afraid you are, you can do this. You know you can. And deep down, you know that you will not be judged. What is happening to you is real, it is not rare, and help is out there. Your doctor's office is the best place to start.

What you need to do is very simple: just pick up the phone and call.

I was lucky enough to have a very close relationship with my OBGYN. When I called his office, not only did he get on the phone right away, but he was able to prescribe an initial dose of antidepressants without making me leave the house and drag myself to an appointment. However, the chances are good that you will need to make the trip to a doctor's office and be examined professionally. Do it, no matter how hard it is. If you can't do it alone, call your partner or a friend and ask them to drive you. Remember that no matter how alone you feel, help and support are just in front of you. All you need to do is reach out.

SOS #4: Opening Up With Family Members

I was diagnosed with Postpartum Depression in early October, and I had been on antidepressants for just two weeks or so when Will's parents came to visit over Halloween. I was not ready to be open at all. I was so ashamed. Here I was, married to their son, the boy they loved so much, and I was a wreck, unable to go a single day without crying.

Amazingly, Will's mom was completely understanding and totally supportive. I had expected her to be uncomfortable about my condition. When I started crying from the shame of needing to take my antidepressant pill, what she said was, "It's okay."

"It takes time," she told me. "You're going to have good days and bad days, you're going to cry. It's not going to get better overnight, but it will get better."

How deeply it struck me when she said that! My mother was not there to hold my hand, but I still needed a mom to tell me that everything would be all right. Far from judging me, my mother-in-law offered me her open heart. It meant the world to me.

Just a few weeks later, we were planning to visit my father's house for Thanksgiving, as we did every year. It was our tradition. I wanted everything to be easy, normal, and happy. But as the holiday approached, I realized that I just couldn't handle making the trip. I was overwhelmed with the mere thought of packing, let alone how I would nurse Brayden, feed Zackery, and take care of the million tiny things that I normally would have taken in stride. The thought of going through with the trip was enough to send me into a panic. We were not going to be able to go.

It had been awkward enough to tell my dad that I had been diagnosed with Postpartum Depression. Even when I did tell him, I never really explained how bad things were. Now I was going to have to tell him that we were breaking our family's beloved tradition. Why? Because I didn't want to come—no, because I couldn't come. It felt incredibly selfish. What I did not understand at the time was that, by saying "no" to Thanksgiving dinner, I was saying "yes" to myself: giving myself permission to be less than perfect, so I could heal. At the time, though, I felt like a terrible daughter who was letting her family down.

Dad was disappointed, and at first he told me, "Let's see how you're feeling next week, maybe you'll change your mind." But I knew that I couldn't make the trip. Frustrated and backed into a corner, I had to open up to him, letting him know how difficult things were for me and that I was just not strong enough.

I don't know what I thought would happen if I disappointed my dad. It's not like he was going to cut me off from the family! But on some level, it felt that way. What really happened was the opposite. Because I opened up and was vulnerable with him, our relationship actually got stronger. He saw a new side of me, different from the strong, stubborn woman I had always shown him. Since then, my dad has shown me some of his vulnerability and compassion, and I have found myself connecting with him on a more emotional level. In the end, it did not matter at all, and I gained the space to heal.

Everyone's family is different, and every relationship has a history that cannot be ignored. Just because you have always related to somebody in a certain way, it does not mean your relationship won't develop and grow. I can't tell you how best to talk to your own family, but I can tell you that it is worth it to try.

For me, opening up and becoming vulnerable brought out a whole new level of compassion from my family, and a new way for me to see them as loving supporters. For you, perhaps they will applaud your strength in seeking help, or support your decision to take medication or pursue other healing methodologies. Our families often see us very differently from how we see ourselves, and if you are lucky, your family will be able to see when you are doing the right thing for your own health and happiness.

SOS #5: Sharing With Acquaintances and Strangers

Once you have accepted the truth of what is happening to you, once you are getting treatment and you have some support from the people closest to you, then it becomes time to choose what you will tell the people you don't know as well. This is an intensely personal choice, but of course I will advise you to be open and honest about your experience. For me, this has been one of the most healing choices of my entire journey.

Before you talk about it, make sure you are talking to the right people. For example, how do you feel in your mommy group or other activities? Some groups (and many moms) can be a bit competitive and drawn to one-upmanship: "Oh, little Johnny had his first smile today," and "Oh, my Maria just sat up on her own." That may not be an environment where you naturally want to share what is going on. You need to find an environment that is safe and supportive.

Brayden's mommy group was just what I needed. They were real, sharing challenges and creating an atmosphere of comfort.

There was no competitiveness at all. Although we pushed each other to grow and succeed, it was always with love and understanding; when I finally admitted that I was taking antidepressants, they could not have been more supportive.

I eventually came to question why I had been hiding my real feelings from these women, when they actually took it completely in stride. Why was I afraid to tell them that I was hurting? The truth was that my pressure to be perfect came from me, and not from them. That is how it should be, if you've got the right people around you!

Eventually, you may find that you're ready to talk openly about your struggles—on social media, at your job, or, like me, very publicly. If you get to this stage, you might be surprised at the reactions you get. When I started talking about PPD on my Facebook page, I heard from women who had never shown any outward signs of depression, but who told me that the last few years had been the darkest time in their lives. "You're not alone, and it gets better," was the overwhelming reaction from these women.

I still meet fellow PPD survivors all the time. Their message is one of love, strength, and hope. So different from the judgment and scorn I had imagined! Not a single person has been unkind or judgmental with me. Not one.

What Will You Say?

I cannot make it any more clear: it is time to speak up, to share your pain, and to ask for help. By now, you know something about what is happening to you, and you know that what you're going through is real and not your fault. You are ready, right now, to pick up the phone and call someone for support.

I know how frightening that is—believe me, I know to the very core of my soul. That is why I am offering you some prompts that might help you figure out how to talk about what is happening. You don't need to fill out all of these. You might not need any of them. But if you still can't find the words, try writing them down here. Then, when it's time, all you need to do is read them off the page.

What I want to say to my partner:

_____

_____

What I want to say to my best friend:

_____

_____

What I want to say to my mom and dad:

_____

_____

What I want to say to my doctor:

_____

_____

Reclaim the Joy of Motherhood

Finally, you might want to explain to your friends and family what you are feeling, and what you are going through. Please use the rest of this space to share your thoughts.

What did you think motherhood was going to be like? What is the reality, and how is it different?

_____

_____

_____

_____

_____

_____

_____

_____

CHAPTER ELEVEN

The Other Side of the Story: How PPD Affects Friends & Family

*"Deep in my heart I'm concealing things that
I'm longing to say*

Scared to confess what I'm feeling

Frightened you'll slip away."

- Evita

❦

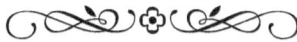

You might think that something so personal and internally emotional as Postpartum Depression would only affect the person going through it. Unfortunately, that isn't true. Postpartum Depression has side effects that impact more than just the individual who is suffering. For me, it affected my relationships with Will, my father and sister, my friends, and even the way I treated myself. It saddens me to think about it, but it also affected my relationships with my children, Zackery and Brayden.

Whether you personally are struggling, or know somebody who is, you know it is a confusing and difficult experience to have a successful relationship through the cobwebs of depression.

Reclaim the Joy of Motherhood

In this chapter, I'm going to share my own story of how PPD affected my relationships, and I'll also share stories from my husband, Will, and my friends, Elisa and Courtney. My hope is that both women with PPD, and the people who love them, will see a little of themselves in these stories, and will grow to understand and support each other even more.

What It Felt Like for Me

When we first brought Zackery home from the hospital, we received many phone calls to see how we were doing. I remember feeling bad that it had taken me so long to get back to people. It wasn't necessarily that I didn't want to talk to them; I just didn't have the time between nursing, sleeping, and trying to figure out this new little being we had brought home with us. Most people understood and were accommodating to my new schedule. I had visitors over at the house and I enjoyed the company.

After Brayden was born, I went through the same dilemma with people calling to see how we were doing, but this time I rarely called them back at all. I kept telling myself, "They'll call again, I'll talk to them later," when really I was hoping they wouldn't. I didn't want to talk to anyone. I didn't want to be bothered. I wished instead that Will would talk to them, run interference for me, and give an update as to how Brayden and I were doing.

I was never one of those girls who spent hours in her room, lying on the bed with her feet up the wall, talking on the phone with the cord twirled around her finger. In fact, I was quite the opposite: I hated talking on the phone—to anyone.

Unfortunately, this was precisely what I needed to be doing.

There were a few, select mommy friends, such as Courtney whom I saw on a regular basis, mostly at the breastfeeding and baby-and-me classes, but also sometimes at play dates or for coffee. There was also my best friend Elisa, who lived about thirty minutes away. None of these women knew what was happening to me. I put on a pretty face, pretending to be happy and "fine," when in reality I was far from it. Who knows if any of them suspected something might be wrong, but they sure didn't hear anything other than "life is good—hard, but good" from me.

Elisa would call, and although I can't recall exact conversations, I think back and realize how one-sided they were. She talked, I listened—as best I could through the fog and cotton balls stuffed in my brain. I didn't have much to say except the same old thing: "I'm tired." This had probably been going on far longer than I realized, likely for the three years I had depression but didn't know it yet.

They say we often hurt the ones we love the most. Will was the one person in my life (aside from Brayden) who was with me more than anyone else. He should have been the first person I confided in, the first person I told that I was scared and ashamed, angry and sad. He should have been the first person I asked for help, but he wasn't. Will, my husband, whom I loved more than anyone, and still do, was one of the last to know. I didn't know how to tell him. I was badly hurting and embarrassed, and didn't want to show my weakness. I was a strong woman, and this shouldn't be happening. I didn't want to burden Will with my pain, and I felt guilty for having to.

I didn't intentionally hurt Will, it just slowly and unconsciously happened. I put a great deal of distance between us as I became more and more withdrawn, eventually losing all closeness. Intimacy after childbirth with two little boys in the house had understandably become challenging. Throw in a little, or rather a lot, of Postpartum Depression, and all desire for any kind of physical contact went flying out the window.

Will always was, and still is, good at taking the boys out and about: to the "green" park to throw rocks in the creek, up the street for a walk, or to the meadow road to ride bikes. Zackery and Brayden have always been blessed with a father who does things with them. What they did not always have is a mother who did the same.

When Zackery and Brayden were younger, when I was in the thick of my Postpartum Depression, I didn't want to do anything. The hikes I used to enjoy and look forward to—they were too troublesome. The park where I could watch the boys go down the slide, or push them on the swings—that was too hard. Everything seemed overly burdensome and difficult, on top of the fact that I just did not want to do anything. I would much rather stay in my pajamas, which I did, day in and day out, even though Zackery and Brayden were dressed.

It got to the point where I couldn't even leave the house unless I was by myself. It was too much for me to take even one of the boys with me. I only took both of them with me somewhere if it was absolutely necessary, like to their own dentist or doctor appointments, or if it was a dual play date at a friend's house with kids the same age. I stopped going to the grocery store unless it was at night, once the boys were asleep in bed and Will was home from work. Funny, that actually became my weekly sanctuary: the grocery store, the place I went to get away.

I lost all energy and desire to do anything fun with the boys. We stayed home—a lot. I skipped the music classes, the gym time, and the playgroups that weren't at a friend's house. I have never believed in over-scheduling children with all sorts of activities, and part of my decision to stay home was based on that, not to mention not having any money to pay for activities. However, even if we weren't too busy and could afford it, my depression held me back from wanting to go.

When I stopped enjoying the activities that once brought me joy, I stopped fully participating in my children's lives. I still feel guilty about that. There is a place in my heart that feels broken for having robbed Zackery and Brayden of those special moments and memories.

The relationship with my father and sister suffered as well. Before kids and before Will, my sister and I were very close. We talked all the time, traveled together, cried and laughed together. Once I had a family of my own, I didn't see my sister as much. I had a husband and two boys at home, but she still just had her career. My circumstances changed and we were now in two different places in life. No judgment, just different.

I never really did talk to my dad or sister about my Postpartum Depression. It wasn't something I felt comfortable sharing with them, even though they were family. They always knew me as a strong, smart, stubborn woman. That woman was the only one I had ever shown them. To now show my weakness and expose my soul to them made me very uncomfortable, so I didn't.

I remember when I finally did tell Will about my diagnosis, calling upon the small amount of courage I somehow found within me. He told me he was actually relieved, not that I had Postpartum Depression, but that it was something that could be diagnosed and treated. To him, being diagnosed with depression explained a lot. It explained everything he saw in me that I didn't see for myself until later: the drastic changes in behavior; the sadness; the crying; the mood swings and irritability; the inability to focus, make a decision, or sometimes even discuss anything; and the anxiety and lack of confidence he witnessed in regards to caring for our boys. I can see how he could have felt relieved with my diagnosis.

It took me a long time to be able to talk to him about my depression. Even now I sometimes find myself being reserved in our conversations. Will has been nothing but supportive, loving, and caring. I honestly don't know what I would have done without him. He gave me space when I needed space, and he gave me security and encouragement when I needed that. More than anything, he understands that my Postpartum Depression took a part of who I was and that I am still rebuilding myself. His patience and unconditional love has probably been the one part of our relationship that never faltered.

Once I felt secure in disclosing my Postpartum Depression and the medication I was now taking, my friends were nothing but supportive, every single one of them. It brought an instant sense of relief to me that they would still accept me, even though I was broken. My load felt lightened and although I still felt uneasy, I knew if I accidently let a tear fall in front of them it would be okay.

I have continued to share with them, and try to remain as open as possible. Most of them know my story, at least the basics of it, and the shame of talking about it no longer haunts me. The last thing I want is for one of my friends to feel the way I did, and be ashamed to express herself.

Today, I'm happy to say my dad and I have regained some of our bond. When I was growing up, we were never really that close, but since becoming an adult I found myself connecting with him on a more emotional level. I'm sure that's part of a natural progression, and common for many father-daughter relationships. He has shown me some of his vulnerability and compassion, which makes it easier for me to open my heart and share with him. He is a loving father who cares about me very much.

I mentioned that my Postpartum Depression also affected the relationship I had with myself. The change that happened within me was a cycle. I went from trying to prevent something I felt I was at risk of, to denial, to awareness, to acceptance, to complete vulnerability in asking for help, to understanding, to beginning to heal, to ultimately where I am now: happy.

I had to get angry with myself for allowing it to happen to me, and I had to forgive myself for not knowing it was something I couldn't control. I had to learn patience with myself, to heal at my own pace, and I had to learn to recognize when I was pushing myself too hard or too fast. I had to let go of the guilt that I did anything wrong, and the guilt of how I had affected so many people around me.

In the end, I found a passion inside me to help others, and this would not have been born if I had not experienced what I did. I have changed. I am not the person I was before, and I am thankful.

What It Felt Like for Others

WILL

My wife's PPD affected me very severely. I knew other new dads whose wives stepped into the mommy role and really took on the whole burden. Now, some of those dads really should have been helping out more. I'm a 50/50 type of guy, I like to think. One new mom said she got up every night, every time, and let her husband sleep because he made the money in their household and needed to rest for work. "As the stay-at-home mom, the babies and getting up at night are my jobs," she said. I was BLOWN AWAY by that.

When Pam first found out her mom was sick, she became very scared and it changed her. I thought to myself, If this is how she is reacting to her mom being sick, I'm not sure Pam will be able to handle it when her mom dies. This was the beginning of when I saw changes in her.

When Pam's mom died, I was actually surprised at how well she was handling it. Before this, I did not know if I would able to be supportive enough. I even had doubts that our marriage would be able to withstand it.

Looking back, I don't think Pam ever fully dealt with the death of her mom. When Zackery was born, we both did not work for three months, so I was there doing a lot of work around the house, and able to help with the baby. I think my being home helped ward off the PPD. I also think Pam focused on Zack and put off grieving for her mom.

She was always very tired and had no energy to do anything. If she took one shower per week, she was doing well. Her ears were constantly ringing, her head hurt, and her hair hurt. She had no motivation to do anything. She did not want to get dressed, did not want to leave the house. It was also one of the 20-year winters in Truckee, and at one point we could not see out of the back of the house because there were eight feet of snow blocking the windows. This is depressing to most people, so I can only imagine the negative effect it had on Pam at the time.

When Brayden was born, she had to stop working, stay at home full time, care for a baby and a two-year-old mostly by herself, worry about money, and not have any family close by or her mom to talk to for help and guidance. I was making a big career change as well, which was very scary for me and possibly for Pam, too. On top of all this, we had maxed out all of our credit and finally had to stop paying our mortgage in order to afford our monthly bills, such as heat, power, and food. I think this all may have culminated into the perfect storm for her to slip into PPD.

COURTNEY

We met while we were both preggers, and our friendship was new, and Pam already had Zack. I took a lot of cues from her about newborns and birth and all that. Once we had the babies, I kind of assumed that we would have similar experiences with our newborns, and in some ways we did—but in others we didn't. That's the first thing I remember. I had trouble breastfeeding—getting my baby to do it—and while Pamela breastfed fine, she had all that thrush to deal with. I remember her telling me one time that she was trying to feed Brayden while potty training Zackery, and that blew my mind. I couldn't imagine that. So, from my point of view, dealing with the thrush, another small child, and other problems that I knew bothered her, it all seemed overwhelming. I didn't know how she was going to handle it all. But at first she did seem pretty in control, or at the very least, up for the challenge.

It wasn't until the babies were getting older and I started to feel like I was getting into the swing of things that I started to notice that Pam was still struggling. And again, with everything she had on her plate, it made sense. I didn't feel like I had the experience to really understand what she was going through and how hard it "should" be.

WILL

After Brayden was born, Pam definitely was not the same. She was very tired and had a challenging time doing much of anything. I was working and also studying for my licenses, and did not have much extra time to help her. I was able to recognize that Pam needed someone to talk to, so I would call our doula or a friend to come and check on her. I didn't think she had PPD, just the normal Baby Blues, I guess, but she was definitely not herself.

ELISA

I remember getting a call from Will asking me to talk to Pam because she was always crying and was having a hard time. That was the first that I had heard about her having a hard time. We did not live close by and I had not heard from her in a while, so I didn't think anything of it, just thought she was hunkering down with the new baby.

When I called Pam, she immediately started to cry. I thought it was post-baby hormones and pretty much told her to "mommy up" and to go to the doctor to get blood work for her hormones if she thought it was that bad. She was very distant in our conversation, and really did not tell me how she was truly feeling. She was very short, and snapped at me. I could tell that everything I was saying, and the advice I was giving her, was not being registered and she was just "yes"ing me.

When I hung up the phone, I thought to myself, Why am I giving advice and trying to help when she doesn't want it? It made me so frustrated. I thought Pam just didn't want to talk to me because she didn't want to hear what I had to say. I NEVER thought it was PPD, and to be honest, I never really believed PPD was considered an illness.

My lame thinking was: You have a baby, it is hard, and you deal with it. Your hormones go out of whack, and when they go back to normal you start to feel better. To treat it like an illness never crossed my mind.

WILL

When I started my new job, I needed to be working 10 to 12 hours per day—but I had to ease into that little by little, to ramp Pam up to being able to manage things with me gone. I almost failed at my job, and could probably name several reasons for that, but I prefer to think that I timed my success as perfectly as I could without either of us, Pam or I, having to default to Plan C.

I thought I understood what she was going through, but now I really don't think I did. What I was feeling was not understanding, more empathy, I guess. But I was supportive in the best way I knew how to be. I just tried to help out by doing as much as I could when I was home.

COURTNEY

There was a point in time when I came across a few things that made me think of Pam. Talking with a friend about her own depression, she explained that she knew she had an issue when there were no happy days. She was always down, and she learned that was a sign. I remember talking to Pam, and she admitted she wasn't having good days. They were all kind of bad, and some days seemed worse.

I also remember watching some talk show about PPD, and how it only used to be discussed when something tragic happened, so women felt uncomfortable talking about it because it had such a horrible connotation. But when they described what mild PPD was, it made me wonder if this was something Pam should look at.

Then Pam started to make flippant comments about "feeling crazy," or "out of control," like she "couldn't take much more of it." That worried me. Pam and I both had the same doula, Marlena, and around that time she asked me what I thought about how Pam was doing. We talked a little about being worried about her.

Within a few days, I think, Pam told me about the night she felt like she was having a heart attack, and how when she looked it up online she could relate to every symptom of PPD.

Marlena talked to Pam and told her to go to the doctor, and then Pam called me. I remember feeling like I was close enough to her to be honest, and that she was ready to move forward. The next step, as scary as it was, was to call the doctor. At the time, from my point of view, I felt like there really wasn't anything to lose. But I do remember praying that he took Pam seriously—because if he didn't, if he left her feeling like she was making it up, that would have put her in a very bad place.

WILL

When Pam called me and asked me to pick up a prescription for her, and then told me it was for PPD, my first thought was YES! Excitement that she was getting help! As soon as she told me she thought she had PPD and had had it since Zack was born, I said, "You're absolutely correct!" I hadn't seen it until that moment, but when she brought it to my attention I could only agree one hundred percent. I was actually happy that something was wrong, that this wasn't her true self. She was not herself because of an illness, and she could now figure out how to start the recovery process. Like anything else, a plan to move forward can only begin once you have stopped and figured out what your current situation is.

ELISA

It was not until later, when she started taking medication, that Pam expressed to me how bad it had been. Not until we were really able to sit down and talk about how she felt did I understand that PPD is a very serious illness. After talking with Pam, and hearing how she did not want to get out of bed or see anyone, I felt so bad and was so sorry I had not been there for her in the way that she needed me.

COURTNEY

This whole thing was surreal for me, because so much of my life at the time was new and different: new baby, new friends, new town… I wasn't totally sure of my opinion of things, but once

Pam got some help and started on the path to help herself—once I got to see her as she really is—then I realized how much it was affecting her. I realized that I hadn't yet really seen her true personality. That left an impression on me.

ELISA

Today, Pam is a completely different person. She sees light and happiness, but she works at it every day and makes time for self-healing. I do believe, now that I understand the struggles she went through, it is easier for her to talk to me at the times when she is scared that she will spiral down to PPD again. I also feel like I understand those feelings and can help by just listening, offering a shoulder to cry on, or giving advice when asked. I am so proud of Pam, and so happy that I get to be a part of the healing process. The struggles will always be there, but Pam is STRONG and I admire her for being able to get her story out to other women.

SECTION III

Reclaiming My Hope & Happiness

CHAPTER TWELVE

Day By Day

*"Far away there in the sunshine are my highest aspirations.
I may not reach them, but I can look up and see their beauty,
believe in them, and try to follow where they lead."*

- Louisa May Alcott

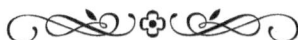

It took so much strength and bravery to make that one decision: to call my doctor and ask for help. It was a big victory, and I am proud of myself for doing it; but once I had made my decision, things did not magically get better right away. I still had a long road of recovery ahead of me. The sky was still dark, and I had a long way to go. The difference, now, was that I was no longer lost. Ahead of me somewhere, happiness was waiting. All I had to do was keep moving toward it, step by step and day by day.

The first few days seemed to bleed into one another as I listlessly survived each moment, not knowing or caring about anything at all. I focused on Brayden, on holding him close to my aching heart, as if his purity and innocence might somehow trickle into my soul and wake me from this nightmare.

It was early October when I was diagnosed with Postpartum Depression, and over the next several weeks I focused on taking a tiny little pill each day, waiting for the magic of happiness in my life. I knew the effects of the antidepressants wouldn't be immediate, but I struggled with patience. I had done the hardest thing possible to me at the time. I had made the call. I had asked for help. So why wasn't I feeling any better? Why did tears still stream down my face? Why couldn't I smile or laugh? Why wasn't I overjoyed with motherhood like I had expected myself to be—like I was supposed to be? Why was I still so, so sad?

Every day, somebody—whether it was Will, or Courtney, or my doula—would ask me the same question. I heard it over and over, like a scratched old 45-rpm record. Sometimes that record would skip to the end, and sometimes it would get stuck in one spot, but it always played the same music, always that familiar refrain: "How are you doing today? Are you feeling all right?" My answer, like the record, was always the same: "I'm okay."

I kept all my thoughts and feelings tightly locked up inside. I hoped that by not sharing my truth, my loitering misery and grief, I could avoid talking about it. The worst, most unpleasant and torturous thing I could imagine was talking about it. I was already suffering. I didn't need or want to add to the pile of gloom that I was buried under. I wanted to break free of this suffocating weight, but I didn't know how.

If and when you start taking antidepressants, your doctor will tell you that they may not work right away—that you may even get worse before you get better. This was the case with me. At first, I just felt lost in the same fog that had enveloped me. I held onto my routine: taking care of Brayden, going to my breastfeeding class and my mommy group. I had a few private conversations with trusted people about what was happening to me, but for the most part I was just surviving, still hiding the turmoil that raged in my heart. I had descended into a place that I could not imagine ever coming back from: a deep black hole, inside the devil's pocket. All I had was one tiny little light: my angel baby, Brayden. No matter what, I was not going to let him down. So I took my pill, and kept up with my tasks, and survived.

Then, one day, I smiled. Not just a formality or scripted reaction, but a genuine, heart-felt smile. Through the fog of memory, I don't recall what caused it, but I do remember that, in that moment, I started to feel hope. Something I had completely given up on ever feeling again.

Hope didn't return to me all at once. It wasn't a beautifully wrapped gift dropped down on me with a thud. It trickled in, like water carving its destined path through granite boulders, and with the same silent power. I drank deeply, treasuring every drop. I hadn't realized how much I needed it.

For a full month, I took my pills and I held my baby and I survived on that trickle of hope. I was still crying often, and I was still tired, insecure, and scared. My husband, family, and friends continued to wrap me in the warmth of their care and support, and they kept asking—"How are you doing today?" One day in November, I realized that my answer had changed from "okay" to "better." I was starting to feel a noticeable difference.

It was another month before I started to toy with the idea of opening up and talking about my story. I knew from past experience that, whatever pain or agony I was going through, it seemed to dissipate more quickly the sooner I gave in and spoke up. The idea still frightened me. I still felt fragile and ashamed, broken and small. I still felt like hiding from reality. Sharing would be hard; hiding was easy. Neither scenario was something I looked forward to. Either one could bring me discomfort, turmoil, and shame. Sharing would mean exposing myself to a place of vulnerability and weakness. Hiding meant that I might not heal, and that no one ever had to know just how far I had gone.

I allowed myself to feel terrified. I acknowledged the fear I would be facing. But this time, instead of reacting to fear by shutting down my emotions, I accepted the journey of healing. It began with conversations: talking openly with Will, Elisa, Courtney, and other close friends and family about what I had gone through and what I was feeling. Then I began sharing my story with the women in my baby-and-me group. The more I shared, the more love and support I received. It was not even close to the shame and judgment I had expected. And although sharing and opening up left me totally vulnerable, it did not make me weak. On the contrary, it was powerful in the love it inspired. Instead of being alone, I discovered that I was surrounded by people who cared deeply, who empathized and tried to understand, and who would support me no matter what. Day by day, with the support of people who loved and cared for me, I began to heal myself.

All my life, I have been a perfectionist and a planner. Before PPD, I had always held firm to the idea that you set a goal, and you achieve it—anything less is a failure. I had always relied on nobody but myself, firmly believing that I could and should be able to do whatever I set my mind to, without help. Asking for help would be weakness, and that would be unacceptable.

Postpartum Depression destroyed that part of me, dismantling my superwoman ego and leaving me completely helpless and weak. And as I rebuilt myself, I found that the old pieces didn't fit into the same configuration. Some of them didn't fit at all. But it didn't matter; the new me is far stronger and more whole than the old me had ever been.

Now, I am no longer controlled by a need to be perfect and independent. That person is gone, and my new self is so much better: Pamela Zimmer, a strong and intelligent woman who has a big heart and cries sometimes, and isn't afraid to show it.

My support system is so much stronger now, too—but it only works if I allow myself to be vulnerable. Elisa and Will are like a couple of coaches now. They talk to each other about how I am doing, and when I slip back into my old habits, they boss me around:

"Come on, Pam, let's get out of the house."

"Pam, you are working too hard, take yourself to the spa this week."

I never would have asked for people to do this for me— independent, self-sufficient me could never have imagined I might need it—but they are my saving grace again and again. The two of them look out for me, catch the signs of overwhelm, and help me stay on track.

Reclaim the Joy of Motherhood

Don't think for a split second that things are "solved" in my life. My depression marked me deeply, and I am still recovering. It is still, and always will be, incredibly hard for me to open up and ask for help, or to accept it when it is offered. That is just who I am, and it is something I will continue to work on every day for the rest of my life. I will always work on being more present and aware of my feelings and my body; and I will always have to fight to take care of myself first instead of putting my health on the back burner.

The difference, now, is that I understand the reality of just how good and how bad things can be. All the demons that I imagined, the pretended consequences of my imperfection, were just puppets created by my own mind, putting on a macabre play to frighten me into submission. The real danger is far, far worse than what those fears threatened: If I do not take care, I can sink down again into the depths of depression, falling back into the devil's pocket where nobody can pull me out again. On the other hand, if I just take care of myself—day by day—then I can feel joy and freedom. I can laugh with my boys, love with my husband, live my life to the very fullest.

It all comes down to what I do, day by day. And so, I stay on the path. I do not wander back into the woods. I am careful, and I don't walk alone. With my friends and family beside me, I continue on toward the ever-brighter horizon and the dream of joy that unfolds before us.

CHAPTER THIRTEEN

Journey To Joy

"The most difficult thing is the decision to act, the rest is merely tenacity. The fears are paper tigers. You can do anything you decide to do. You can act to change and control your life; and the procedure, the process is its own reward."

- Amelia Earhart

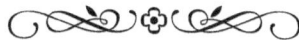

My recovery may be ongoing, but it is also very successful. I feel happier all the time; friends and acquaintances are always telling me how much I have changed; my family has grown closer; and my ability to stay on track has improved by leaps and bounds. I never could have begun to heal without the help of my friends, Will, and my doctor; but they could not do the work of healing for me. That was something I needed to learn on my own, and I think I've done it!

I want the same feeling for you. I want all women who are struggling with Postpartum Depression to have a path toward happiness that they can follow. To that end, I have developed a mentorship program that offers new ideas to try, tips for staying on track, and support to keep moving forward. I call it

The HAPPY Mommy Method™, and it is designed to accompany medical treatment, to help women like you recover faster and more fully.

In this chapter, I want to give you the most important piece of The HAPPY Mommy Method™, so that you can begin to put it into practice in your own life. Here, you will find the five steps that make up the healing process. I'll share with you how I followed each of these steps, and give you ideas to try in your own life. My hope is that this chapter will be your guide to recovery, and that you will turn back to it often.

1. Find a Trust Person

The first thing you must do is something that we have talked about before: Find somebody who makes you feel safe, in whom you can put your trust. It doesn't necessarily need to be your doctor; it might be a close friend or your doula, or a family member. It just needs to be someone you feel comfortable with, who won't judge you, and to whom you can talk with honestly and regularly.

I've told you about my two trusted confidantes: my doula Marlena, and my friend Courtney. They were the first ones I felt I could talk with openly, and they provided me with just the help I needed.

When choosing your trust person (or people), be very aware of the way they make you feel when you share your struggles. There is an important difference between a person who listens to you, and a person who supports you.

"I see many women minimizing what another woman is going through, saying 'This is motherhood, it's hard, just hang in there'," says Kristin Hodson, founder of The Healing Group. "There is a belief that motherhood is hard, that we've all been in the trenches and to just hunker down and get through. While motherhood is challenging, motherhood doesn't mean you need to suffer." If you find that the person you are opening up to is not fully supportive of your need for extra help, seek another source of support.

Who can you trust and be open with right now?

_____

How often do you talk to this person?

_____

Do you feel supported when you talk to this person? Why or why not?

_____

Is there anyone else in your life in whom you would like to confide?

_____

2. Find an Outlet

Part of healing from emotional turmoil is learning not to deny your feelings. They are too powerful! If you try to shut them down, you will often fail, or spend a lot of energy fighting your body's natural process. Rather than trying to hold back the tides, you can find a way to channel them so they do not cause destruction in your life. You can even find ways to make your feelings have positive influence, instead of negative.

For me, writing was my outlet. I have always been a writer at heart. Writing has come easily and naturally to me, and it has consistently been my means of communication whenever emotions are high or life is tough.

It was always obvious to me that I would eventually write about my depression. What I did not expect was the difficulty of writing down the dark, demonic images and thoughts that were still encircling my heart. At times, I was afraid to write, for fear of experiencing those horrible, unwanted thoughts again. Other times, I didn't even know what to write. I would stare at my computer, my mind as blank as the screen. Eventually, I had to give in and let the words flow, no matter how evil they seemed or how dangerous they looked. I had to release all the demons, or they would continue to consume me.

I know now that the process of creating something from your pain is an important part of healing. It works on a subconscious level that is difficult to understand or explain. Once I let the demons fly free, my heart was cleared of some of the darkness. And on the page, the demons do not look as large as they feel when they're in your blood.

Your outlet can be anything that you do when you need a break or an escape from the pressure. It should not be unlawful or unhealthy, such as alcohol or drugs. It should not be something that becomes compulsive or addictive—no running ten miles without eating, please! Instead, your outlet should be something that fills your heart with joy. It should be fun, never an obligation, but a gift to yourself.

Your outlet can be anything you choose. Here are some ideas:

- Writing or journaling
- Meditation
- Prayer
- Yoga
- Walking
- Other fun exercise
- Singing
- Dancing
- Making music
- Cooking
- Painting
- Drawing
- Sewing

What are some things that you love doing for fun?

_____

_____

_____

_____

3. Consistent Care

This is where your doctor or care provider comes in. If you want to recover and heal on every level, you must combine self-care strategies with qualified medical guidance. So, you need to keep up with your appointments and medication (if applicable), and keep an eye on your symptoms.

Some women will not need medication, and some will take it for the rest of their lives. Many, like me, will struggle with it at first, then find that it helps tremendously, and eventually learn other strategies in order to live without it.

Some women do not enjoy talk therapy, and some love the opportunity to see the "brain doctor" for clues as to what is happening with their mental chemistry. Some will try more than one counselor before finding a person we respond to and connect with.

Your care plan is up to you and your doctor, and it will be completely different from person to person. The only thing we all have in common is that we need to be consistent about our treatment. If you have an appointment, go. Update your doctor and/or therapist about what is happening with you. Let them treat you to the best of their ability.

When was your last doctor's appointment? Do you need to go in again soon?

_____

_____

_____

_____

Are you taking medication? How is it working?

_____

_____

_____

_____

Do you need or want an adjustment in your medication?

_____

_____

_____

_____

Have any of your symptoms been getting better or worse? How?

_____

_____

_____

_____

Do you have any new symptoms to talk to your doctor about?

_____

_____

_____

_____

4. Consistent Daily Routine

When you are healing, your life is a balancing act. A little misstep can make you feel like you are completely out of control. So, the best thing you can do for yourself is to be consistent. Do the little things that make your life run smoothly, and do them on a schedule that works for you without stress.

It is also important for your baby to follow a routine. Babies thrive on consistency, as they adjust to all the sensory input and unexpected events of life outside the womb. Just by creating patterns and habits, you can help your child feel safe and happy from day to day.

For me, the routine was what kept me going between my diagnosis and the time when I really started to feel strong again. When I felt weak, it was okay, because I still had my routine. I knew that, no matter what, I was taking care of the necessities and doing the things that I believed would make me stronger, eventually. Some days, the necessities were all I could do. No matter what, it felt good to know that I was taking care of myself, and never letting myself down.

Every woman's life and needs are different, so your daily routine might be very different from your neighbor's. Here are some ideas of things you might include on your daily routine list:

- Taking your medication (if applicable) every day, preferably at the same time

- Making time (at least 5-10 minutes) for your outlet every day

- Eating healthy food and drinking plenty of water
- Getting enough rest and nighttime sleep
- Creating a consistent routine for your baby

What are the things you need to do every day for your life to run smoothly?

_____

_____

_____

_____

_____

_____

5. Celebrate!

When you accomplish something, no matter how big or how small, make sure you celebrate it! Giving yourself positive feedback is great for your brain, and it also helps you reinforce those baby steps forward while making the step-by-step process a little less monotonous. You deserve appreciation for making progress. It is not easy, and you're doing it anyway. So celebrate yourself!

Here are some things you might be celebrating:

- Taking your pill
- Drinking eight glasses of water in a day
- Talking with your trust person
- Talking with other friends and family

Reclaim the Joy of Motherhood

- Using your outlet
- Going for a walk
- Taking a nap
- Being consistent with your routine
- Feeling good!

You should celebrate these little accomplishments every day. That's right: Every single day, find something positive to appreciate about yourself. Here are some ways you might celebrate:

- Write down your accomplishment(s) in a gratitude journal
- Tell your trust person
- Talk to your support group
- Give yourself a treat (a pedicure or a new book, a coffee or a piece of pie, but not the whole pie!)

Over time, you will start to see how far you have come, and those little wins will add up to something very big. When that happens, you will see your step-by-step healing process in a whole new way.

- What is something good that you accomplished today?
- Is there anything else that you are happy or proud about recently?

After working through this chapter, you have probably learned some new things about yourself, and I am sure you have some new ideas to try. Remember that recovery, just like everything

150

else, is a process that you can adopt gradually. Do not worry about whether you're doing it "right," but be patient and loving with yourself. Over time, these healthy habits will become just that—habits—and you will continue to find new pathways toward your joy. For now, just focus on today. You have come so far already, and there is still a long road ahead.

CHAPTER FOURTEEN

Finding the Right Treatment

"I read and walked for miles at night along the beach, writing bad blank verse and searching endlessly for someone wonderful who would step out of the darkness and change my life. It never crossed my mind that that person could be me."

- Anna Quindlen

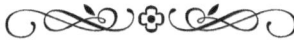

In our beautiful world, every single person is different. From the shape of your toes, to the blood coursing through your veins, to the memories and thought patterns in your brain, you are a unique individual—and nobody, absolutely nobody knows you better than yourself. And yet, for all our uniqueness, each of us eventually finds ourselves in the same spot. No matter who you are or what you have experienced, eventually you will come to a dead end or "rock bottom" with only one way out: asking for help.

"The real threat is not acknowledging one's suffering, but rather continuing to live in pain knowing treatment and relief exist," says Valerie McManus, a social worker and psychotherapist. No matter what is happening with you, once you begin to seek help, you begin moving toward healing. We all make the same choice when we ask for help. We are choosing to survive and get better. But from that simple and clear starting point, our paths diverge greatly. Each of us has a different "me" to get back to, and a different way to get there. What is yours?

In this chapter, I will not advise you on a course of treatment. Though I am an expert on Postpartum Depression, I am not a medical doctor or a trained counselor. While you are working through this book, I also want you to seek out the experts who can give you the personalized approach that will help you find true healing and recovery. So, instead of telling you what to do, I will give you guidelines for your journey. You have a long period of healing ahead of you, and I am proud to support and mentor you through it—but it is your journey to make.

When I work with women who are beginning this journey, I always share the "Golden Rules of Healing," which have guided my recovery and will help you, too.

Be Patient. Extremely, extremely patient. Every single step will take time, often longer than you want to wait. But in time, as long as you are following the Golden Rules, you will heal.

Never Compare. Do not worry about what your friends and neighbors are doing or have done. Everybody's situation is different, and your symptoms can be vastly different, too. What worked for them might not work for you, or it might work on a different schedule. Just focus on your own recovery.

Trust. Trust your choices, trust your instincts, and trust yourself to heal. And trust your doctor or care provider, because when you share what is happening with you, he or she will find the right treatment.

"There is hope," says Kristin Hodson, founder of The Healing Group. "With help and support you will get better. You deserve to feel like yourself again. There is not strength in suffering." Take those words to heart as you begin the process of finding the treatment that will carry you home to your place of joy and health.

Finding the Right Doctor

The first step to truly being able to trust your doctor, of course, is to find a doctor you can trust. For some people, this is easier than for others. I consider myself very lucky to have a great relationship with my OBGYN. When I called and asked for help, he and I discussed all the options right there on the phone. It was a long conversation, and he listened to what I had to say, letting me have a choice in my own treatment. It's so important that you feel able to trust and confide in your own doctor, and that you have some control over your treatment.

If this is not the case for you, you either need to improve your relationship with your doctor, or find a new one. How you go about this, of course, is up to you. Your doctor should respect your feelings and wishes, but for many people, the first step is finding the confidence to be totally honest. You need to share the whole story so your doctor can find the right approach.

If you have opened up and been completely honest with your doctor but still don't feel that he or she is someone you can trust to give you the best treatment, then by all means look for a new doctor. Not everyone in this world is destined to get along, and you have every right to seek out treatment that works for you. This is incredibly important—your happiness is at stake.

Striking Your Own Balance

The two most commonly prescribed forms of treatment are medication and talk therapy. Though these are certainly not your only options, the odds are strong that you will try one or both of these approaches. Exactly how you go about it, however, is up to you and your doctor.

When I had that first tearful conversation with my OBGYN, we spent about half an hour talking about this exact topic. In the end, I felt that medication was the most immediate way to get help. I was resistant to talk therapy: I was ashamed and uncomfortable talking about what was happening to me, so why would I want to go to an office appointment and talk about it some more? Nonetheless, my doctor suggested I try it when I was ready. Yours might tell you something similar. In the end, you don't know what will work until you try.

That does not mean that you should do anything that goes against your beliefs or gut feelings. Some women are totally against taking medication, and I completely support your right to take that stance. Others, myself included, are careful about which medications to take while breastfeeding. If you do not want to take a specific medication, or if you want a lower dose, say so. Ultimately, if taking a pill makes you feel guilty or worried, then it is not helping much, is it?

"While a small amount of antidepressant medication is circulated to an unborn fetus and leached into breastmilk, so are the stress and depression related chemicals including adrenaline, cortisol and norepinephrine," says Valerie McManus. "It has yet to be studied which of these chemical scenarios pose less risk to a fetus or newborn." Scientists simply don't know yet whether it is less harmful for you to breastfeed while taking antidepressants, or to breastfeed while producing high levels of stress chemicals.

"If a risk/benefit analysis shows that the mother would benefit more from taking an SSRI than the potential risk to her baby, then I will recommend she see a medical doctor," says Stacey Glaesmann, a wellness consultant. It is a choice that must be made on a case-by-case basis, and you have every right to make the choice that sits easiest in your heart.

At the same time, if you choose to avoid medication, then you need to become more aware about natural remedies, including how your diet and exercise affect your emotional health. I found an essential oil that really lifts my spirits, and that I can use all day long without worrying about what it is doing to my body. I also work hard to avoid junk food and sweets (which is incredibly hard, and not always successful, thanks to my dangerous sweet tooth).

"I see women recommending all sorts of 'natural' interventions, trying to avoid 'therapy' at all costs," says Kristin Hodson, founder of The Healing Group. "Talk therapy is one of the most natural interventions around. I would love to see mental health and counseling get destigmatized."

Talk therapy, for many people, is a huge help. It is your chance to talk in complete confidence with a trustworthy person who will not judge you, but will listen and help. It is a safe and secret place, and it is completely natural. With my doctor's support and recommendation, even though I wasn't confident it would work, I saw a psychologist.

The experience I took away from my therapy session was validation. I remember her exact words: "Well, no wonder you're depressed." Hearing someone else tell me it was okay to be having the emotions and even the physical sensations I was experiencing—it was what I needed. I was glad to have an "expert" tell me that I hadn't been making it all up.

Ultimately, I just never "clicked" with my therapist. I was lucky, because not only did I have people around me who were openly supportive, but I had another outlet: my writing. I was more comfortable telling my journal about my experience than I was talking to a professional. And so, after giving it a shot, I decided not to continue my talk therapy. Not everyone understood why I was stopping, but I knew that I had been open and patient, had discussed it with my doctor, and had found that it was not right for me.

This is why it is so important to follow the Golden Rules. Everyone's experience is going to be so different. You have to be open and patient, and give things a chance to work. You need to understand that what works for your neighbor might not work for you at all. And you need to trust that, when you and your doctor make a choice about your treatment, it's a good one.

Sticking With It

In the previous chapter, I gave you five steps to the healing process. But the reality is, those are not five steps that you will complete and be done with forever. You will be revisiting them over and over as you move up and down the ladder. The healing process doesn't always move forward, after all. Sometimes you will go backward—even fall down to the bottom again. That does not mean you have failed. You can't fail ever again, because you have a plan and know what you need to do.

Those words probably won't help much when you are feeling bruised and sad, however. You need to create consistent habits and support structures to get you through the hard times. This is exactly why the five steps exist! When you fall, just reach for the nearest rung of the ladder, and begin to pull yourself back up.

When I was diagnosed with Postpartum Depression, I was breastfeeding and intended to continue as long as possible. There really was only one medication my doctor felt was okay for me to try. I started on a 25mg test dose of Zoloft for seven days, to see how my body would react. I didn't experience any of the possible adverse side effects, so my doctor renewed my prescription for the full, thirty-day, 50mg dose.

My doctor told me that it could take a month or more for the medication to start to take effect, and it did. Every day, I took my "happy pill," but for a while I did not feel happier. It was not until November, pretty much thirty days later, that I started to feel the dense fog lift from my mind. I could think, not deeply or consistently, but logical thoughts began to randomly fade in and out. The medication was finally working.

The next month, I felt myself plateau. Then I sensed myself slipping back down into the shadows. It was December. The holidays are hard on many people, and they were hard on me, too. To make things worse, we were completely out of money.
The emotional conflict might be what caused the change, or it might have been my body building up immunity to the medication, or a combination of the two. I was afraid—scared I would be pulled under again.

Thank goodness for my "trust person" (or trust people in this case!). When I told Marlena and Courtney about how I was feeling, they reminded me that my doctor had said this might happen.

"He said that if you felt worse, you should call and let him know," Courtney gently reminded me.

When I did call my doctor, he told me that I probably needed to take a higher dosage. Now my "happy pill" was 100mg instead of 50mg, and from that point forward, it began to work consistently.

I continued to take one little pill each day, until finally I got to the point where it was second nature and part of my daily ritual. I didn't have to keep the sticky note on the bathroom mirror, reminding me to "take your pill." Will didn't have to ask if I took it. We both knew, with confidence, that I was doing what I was supposed to be doing to get better.

If you ever find yourself tempted to give up on your treatment, please, talk to somebody first—especially if you are thinking of stopping your medication. Above all, it is very important that you make a plan for weaning off the medication, instead of stopping cold turkey. "I think what's more harmful than medication side effects," says Kristin Hodson, "is a mother who has been on an anti-depressant consistently, and suddenly goes off the medication without really weighing the pros and cons. It's important to recognize that the health of the mother impacts the health of the baby." Your decisions can make a huge difference in your baby's development; always remember that your ultimate goal is for you both to be healthy and happy.

There is so much relief that comes from having a plan. And yet, there will be many times when you are frustrated and feel like giving up on the recovery process. It will not always be smooth and easy. It will take much longer than you want it to. You and your doctor might make mistakes as you learn and evolve through the process. Whatever you do, just don't give up on those Golden Rules: Be Patient, Never Compare, and Trust.

Journaling

For me and for many women like me, keeping a daily journal is an important part of the emotional healing process. My journal became my voice, and it became the book you are reading right now! I know that not every woman will be compelled to write down every thought and feeling the way I am, but I do strongly advise that you keep a journal, and that you write in it every day.

Your journal is your record of your progress. When your body and mind are going through big changes, it can be difficult to keep track of the details. But your recovery can rely on those details. How are you sleeping? How are you eating? Are you crying more or less? Smiling? Dreaming? All of these things are indicators of your internal changes, and it is very important to track them.

If you have not done it yet, get a journal today. It can be absolutely any format that works for you. In fact, the more comfortable and easy it is for you to use, the better. You want it to be something that you can easily use every day, and work into your daily routine with a minimal effort.

Your journal might be:

- A moleskin notebook
- A sticky note pad
- A text document in a locked folder on your computer
- A voice memo
- A blog
- ...Or anything else you want it to be!

I would tell you that there is no right or wrong way to journal, but that would be a lie. The right way is the way that is comfortable and easy, and that you can do every day. The wrong way makes you uncomfortable, or makes you not want to do it.

When you begin journaling, you might want to follow the prompts below. However, there is absolutely no need to stick to them. You can journal about anything and everything that comes into your head. Fall into the stream of consciousness! You can begin with one thought, and end a million thoughts away. It is healthy, and it is allowed. Speak your mind.

Here are some journal prompts that you might enjoy:

- Did you take your medication (if applicable)? Do you feel any different?

- How did you feel today as opposed to yesterday?

- What made you smile or feel happy today?

- What did you do for yourself today?

- What did you do for your baby today?

- What are you thankful for?

- Did you step out of your comfort zone today?

- Did you eat healthy food today?

- How are you sleeping? Do you dream at night?

Reclaim the Joy of Motherhood

Your journal is just for you; you never need to show it to anybody. However, over time you may notice changes and trends that you will want to share with your doctor, therapist, or trust person. That is a perfect use for this information, but even if you never share a word of what you are writing, you are creating positive change just by opening up mental pathways for your recovery to follow.

The process of healing is deep and intimate. It will teach you so many new things about yourself that you never realized (and maybe that you didn't particularly want to know), but always remember that things are working far, far below the surface. You may not realize that something is changing, but on a subconscious or even chemical level, something amazing might be happening. Give it time, space, and trust. You are on the path, and you will find your way.

CHAPTER FIFTEEN

Daily Happiness Hygiene

"When you find peace within yourself, you become the kind of person who can live at peace with others."

- Peace Pilgrim

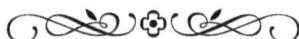

When you begin taking steps to defeat Postpartum Depression, the role of treatment is clear and evident: It is going to make you better. You have been smothered in a dense fog that makes it hard to see or breathe, and you need something or somebody to help lift that fog as soon as possible, just so you can survive. At first, your treatment feels like your only hope in a world that is beyond your control.

Once the suffocating fog begins to break, when you again start to feel the sunlight and breathe the clear air, you may begin to look at your treatment in a new way. For me, while at first taking my medication was an absolute necessity, it eventually became a welcome part of my life. I knew that the pill was working. It was making me feel better, and if I didn't take it, I wouldn't feel better. I was okay with that, and I knew I needed it. Just being able to breathe and think clearly was such an improvement over the past years, and I relied on that pill to keep the clouds away.

After a while, though, I stopped wanting to feel dependent on my antidepressant medication. I wanted to be in control of my happiness again, and to do that, I would eventually have to find another way to keep the fog away. In addition, I have always tried to lead a relatively natural lifestyle. I believed my body could take care of itself without help. Clearly, my old personality was starting to return—my old stubbornness and ambition, which were at odds with the part of me that really needed to surrender, practice patience, and let the treatment work.

After twelve months, I saw my family doctor (who was managing my treatment now that I no longer needed to see my OBGYN) to talk about weaning off my medication. Ironically, I cried throughout the entire appointment. Clearly, as badly as I wanted to take that next step, I was not ready. It really was too soon. Many people stay on their medication for years, and you might even take it for the rest of your life if it works well for you—remember, everyone is different. As for me, I needed a bit more time, and my doctor could see that. She convinced me to keep taking the medication for another six months.

When it was finally time to start cutting back my dosage, Will was really worried for me. We were right in the middle of packing up our home in Truckee so that we could short sell it and move to nearby Reno. We were finalizing our bankruptcy and starting over from scratch. Things were not exactly stable. The last thing Will probably wanted was for me to descend back into depression.

"Why can't you just wait a little longer?" he asked me.

"You know, hon," I said, "all of these problems aren't going to go away just because I take a little happy pill. I have to learn how to handle things that are out of my control."

Once I got Will to understand my perspective, that I wanted a fully clear head to tackle these transitions, he gave me support. I don't believe he agreed with my decision, but he respected that it was my choice, my mind, my body. I felt him keeping a more watchful eye over me, worrying and sometimes even suggesting that I wait—but I didn't, I couldn't. I felt strongly about my choice, and my stubbornness shone through like a sunburst. I had made up my mind, and neither body nor logic could deter me from reaching for the hope I had brewing inside my heart.

Of course, the irony is that in order to reach my new goal of happiness and health, I would need to learn the difference between stubbornness and strength. I would need to develop new skills to help me handle the ups and downs of life. I would not be able to continue treating myself the way I had in the past. The same is true for you, dear reader. How will you take care of yourself now and for the rest of your life?

Developing Your Happiness Hygiene

Once your treatment starts working and the clouds part, you will again be able to breathe deeply and look calmly and logically at the past and the future. At this point, you should start to examine some of the factors that may have contributed to your illness, and how you can potentially avoid the same reaction in the future.

Reclaim the Joy of Motherhood

If you are planning on having more children, you may be worried that PPD will return. "Research shows that there is up to a 75% chance of getting PPD again after a woman has had it once, even if she had several children before experiencing PPD for the first time," says Stacey Glaesmann, a wellness consultant. "Some moms stop after one child if they had a particularly rough time, including myself."

Valerie McManus, a social worker and psychotherapist, has seen that having a strong plan can actually keep future illness at bay. "With the right support and safeguarding, a woman who suffered PPD with her first child has the opportunity to arm herself adequately prior to having subsequent children, thus reducing her risk of relapse. Should she relapse, she may be able to recover more quickly." PPD does not need to limit your options, as long as you are actively practicing happiness.

When I asked my expert sources if there was one common risk factor they had personally observed among women with PPD, they agreed that a "perfectionistic personality" is a big one. "I often see women who have an ideal of what a mother is or should be, trying to walk a rigid line of perfectionism in an effort to be the best mom possible," says Kristin Hodson, founder of The Healing Group. "The pursuit of perfectionism seems to be a common theme among a lot of clients." Personally, I have no doubt that my own perfectionistic goal-setting contributed to my stress and shame when I couldn't "do it all." In order to truly beat PPD, I had to overcome that fundamental part of my personality. Not to make it go away, but to learn how to live with it. That process will probably continue for the rest of my life, and it has become a part of my own happiness program—the things I do to stay sane and keep the fog away.

Your struggle might be something completely different. You might need to gain more confidence, or maybe you need to work on financial stability. Perhaps you have a difficult relationship with the father of your child, or maybe you work too hard. It is different for everyone, and only you can know what needs to change. Look to your trust person and your mentor or therapist (if you have one) for advice. Now you can begin to create a plan that will carry you forward into the rest of your life, free from depression

Keep Doing What Works

This seems obvious, but I know from personal experience that it is easy to stop practicing one of the healthy habits you have spent all this time building, only to see the clouds come crashing back down to suffocate you. Just a few weeks before writing this, I had a terrible week. Looking back, I just want to kick myself—yes, bad things happened that I couldn't control, but I also had not been taking care of myself properly. If I had only stuck with my self-care, I would have been able to handle the week's unfortunate events. Instead, I let them bring me down.

By now, if you have been following through this book (and I hope you have!), you've probably developed a few habits of your own. Maybe it's a weekly coffee with your trust person, or a fifteen-minute nightly journaling time, or a daily "pat on the back" for all your accomplishments. Looking back at your recovery, what are some of the things that fill your soul with sunlight?

169

What habits are working best for you so far?

_____

_____

_____

_____

_____

It is vitally important that you keep up with these rituals and patterns, even as you try new things. Start from here, and begin to add new practices.

The following steps are a continuation of The HAPPY Mommy Method™, which I introduced two chapters ago. Whereas in that chapter we talked about the "process" to begin recovery, now we will talk about your physical health, and about learning to put yourself first.

Take Care Of Your Physical Health

When I first stopped my medication, I was experiencing a lot of strange physical ailments. I had a ringing in my ears that hadn't stopped in two years. My head hurt a lot, and the nerve endings in my face weren't working correctly. Those weren't all the symptoms—lots of little things came and went. I didn't know if they were side effects of the medication, or hormones (which is what everyone kept telling me), or something else. I got tested for everything from thyroid disease to Lyme disease. None of the tests turned up anything.

When I finally stopped the medication, I was able to focus on what was happening with my body. I had learned a lot about breathing through yoga and HypnoBirthing®, and I began taking time to just breathe and be aware and mindful of my body. The more I just listened to my body, the more I understood.

Each of us has a different relationship with her body, but when you are recovering from any illness that has a physical component like Postpartum Depression, it is very important that you get used to being aware of how your body feels. A big part of that is simply breathing deeply.

When you are sad, fearful, tired, or tense, your body also tenses up and you stop breathing deeply. Unfortunately, this can make you feel worse, as your circulation worsens and you are less able to think clearly. This can also worsen any pain you might have. You can't go through life holding your breath, and you would be amazed how well it works to just take two minutes and breathe deeply! When I start to feel stressed and panicky, I take five to ten minutes just to breathe. The rejuvenation and flow I feel is immediate and powerful.

Try it now. In the back of this book, in the Resource Guide, there is a full breathing meditation. I invite you to read through it and give it a try. I believe you will feel so much more relaxed by the end. What a difference five or ten minutes can make.

Aside from breathing, there's another important thing you should be doing. Can you guess what it is? You probably think I'm going to tell you to exercise—but even more important for moms like you and me is rest. You have got to take the time to rest and let your body replenish, not just when you are nursing, but whenever you are taking care of others. Think about it: Do Olympic athletes train all day, every day? Of course not.

They rest, to let their bodies replenish the cells and energy that make them perform at such high levels. If an athlete cannot go-go-go all the time without rest and relaxation, why should you? This is one of the biggest problems in our society: We have an unhealthy feeling that we need to do everything, all the time. Everything needs to be perfect, and we can always work harder—that is absolutely untrue, and it makes us physically unwell, like it did with me.

It turned out that my assortment of bizarre symptoms was most likely linked to adrenal fatigue. I was literally exhausted. After my mother's death, the stress of running and then shutting down my business (not to mention the stress I put on myself to be a perfect mom), the financial trouble, and the daily dramas of raising two small children, I was completely out of energy. My adrenal glands were malfunctioning, and the best thing I could do was simply to sleep, which I did, for what felt like months. It was amazing to give myself permission to rest—a luxury I had never before allowed myself.

Yes, you should exercise too, but make sure you are doing it in a way that feels good and healthy. Make sure that it is improving your life and your state of mind. For many moms, after chasing a child around the house all afternoon, a nice quiet evening walk by yourself is just the ticket. Do what makes you feel healthy.

This also extends to the food you're eating. I've mentioned before that I have a deadly sweet tooth. It can take all my self-control not to eat an entire bag of M&M's—and sometimes I do allow myself to indulge. But most of the time, I take care to eat a balanced diet because I know that junk food and sugar can make your mood run wild. This is even more important when you are so busy that you barely have time to eat. Make sure you do eat, and make sure there's a vegetable in there somewhere. Green is good!

"Research continues to emerge citing the tremendous benefits of a regular meditation or breathing practice, movement and exercise, proper nutrition, methods of self-care, and other practical supports in the resolution of postpartum and other mood disorders," says Valerie McManus. It should not surprise you that when your body feels good, your mind feels good too.

What are one or two things you can do every day to improve or maintain your physical well-being?

_____

_____

_____

_____

_____

Is there anything else about your physical health that you want to work on (e.g. learning to be more aware, getting more rest, etc.)?

_____

_____

_____

_____

_____

_____

_____

Put Yourself First

In airline safety briefings, they tell you that, in case you need to put on an oxygen mask, you should always put yours on first and then help the people around you. Because really, what help can you give if you're unconscious? It may sound silly, but when you are taking care of other people, you should always think of it this way. You have to fill yourself up first, and then you can give everybody else your overflow. Otherwise, you will wear yourself out, and that is no laughing matter.

If you come over to my house right now, I can tell you what you'll probably see: My kitchen counter is going to be a mess. So sue me. I am human, I'm normal, and I have two small boys. We are happy and well-fed, and our kitchen counter is a mess. It's okay. I have learned that, since I have only so much time in a day, I can either focus on cleaning the crumbs, or I can focus on myself and my family. When I look at it that way, the choice is easy.

I also mentioned that I try to eat healthy food. But you know what? Some days, I am too tired to cook. We eat pizza and ice cream for dinner now and then, and I do not feel guilty. I don't even feel guilty when I sleep in an extra fifteen minutes in the morning instead of helping Will make breakfast. I have learned that I really, really need my rest, and that fifteen minutes in the morning will make my entire day run more smoothly.

When I sleep in, or serve up pizza, or neglect to keep my house spotless, I'm actually making a proactive choice. I have learned, over time, that these are the little things that literally could drive me crazy—or I can learn to let them go and find my joy.

Those little rebellions (plus a weekly spa date) keep me happy and sane. They fill me up with light and air, and I float through my days on a warm breeze instead of falling into the fog. You can find your joys, too, and they will be different for everyone. For some of the women I work with, it's an hour spent walking in the morning. Others need to stay up after everyone has gone to bed and the house is quiet. Two chapters back, you started to identify some of the escapes that bring you bliss and peace. I hope you have been practicing them. No matter what, now is the time to begin in earnest. Try to find an escape every single day, so that you are always filled up.

What are some escapes that you know will fill you with happiness?

_____

_____

_____

_____

_____

_____

Physical well-being and putting yourself first are two practices that march hand-in-hand, and if you can keep both of them in motion, you will find that the fog of depression can almost never beat its way past those two soldiers of light. However, keeping up with both practices can be difficult to do. It has taken me five years to learn the balance; if you can get a rhythm going in less time than that, you are doing great.

Reclaim the Joy of Motherhood

One of the best ways to stick with your happiness program is to enlist your trust person, or another confidant whom you see regularly and who you know will look out for you. In my life, I have several people whom I share with; Elisa and Will are the most actively involved. They hold me accountable to my peaceful, happy self. When I am being crabby and complaining too much, they know that it's because I have not been taking care of myself, and they will stop me in my tracks before I run myself right off a cliff. We all need these people in our lives. It can be very hard to give up control and let somebody boss you around, but when Elisa tells me to take a time-out, I listen. I know she sees me for who I am, and I know that sometimes she sees what is happening even better than I do.

Who is one person that will hold you accountable for your happiness?

_____

_____

_____

_____

In the end, nobody but you can truly understand where you are coming from. But that does not mean you are alone, and it does not mean you can't change. In front of you lies your entire lifetime, stretching out to the gilded horizon. There will always be a few clouds: Hard times come and go and you cannot control them, but they cannot obscure your view, suffocate your air, or keep you from continuing on your journey. You have the power to keep them at bay. So breathe deep, smile, and take a spa day.

CHAPTER SIXTEEN

My Passion of Purpose

"Every great dream begins with a dreamer. Always remember you have within you the strength, the patience, and the passion to reach for the stars to change the world."

- Harriet Tubman

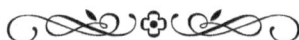

I never really thought anybody would want to read my story. I'm no superstar celebrity, nor have I overcome terrible odds to find success. I wasn't born into tragedy or riches. I'm just a normal person. I have never labored under the delusion that my life was extraordinary, and at first, I honestly did not think of my experience as a "story" that needed telling.

Still, I have always been a writer at heart. Writing has always come easily and naturally to me, and it has been my lifeline whenever emotions are high or life is tough. I enjoy writing, and in many ways it is my outlet. And so in 2010, without any expectation of the result, I created a blog and began filling it with words. This is the first post I wrote about my depression:

Reclaim the Joy of Motherhood

October 2010

Postpartum Depression is real. I have it.

I had it before with my first son (I didn't know it at the time), but this time it has decided to show itself much later, and I believe with more symptoms. It's something I have been aware of (because I had it before) and have tried very hard to keep myself from spiraling down into a depression, but I now know it's not something I can control by myself.

What's hard about believing I have PPD is that at various times throughout the day I feel just fine. What I know, however, is that part of PPD is mood swings – and those I have. I also have many other symptoms – irritability, extreme fatigue, sleeplessness (despite pure exhaustion), crying, lack of desire to do anything (including getting dressed or even brushing my teeth), feeling numb or empty inside. And then there's even the physical symptoms – those I never had the last time. I thought I was having a heart attack the other night when my chest starting hurting as I was nursing my son for the third time in the middle of the night. After much research, I read that chest pain can be a symptom of depression. I was relieved, sort of, that I didn't need to call 911 or go to the hospital for an EKG. But what that made me realize is that I need to get help for my PPD.

Where do I start? Who do I talk to? What do I say? I haven't even told my husband.

I know I shouldn't feel ashamed. But I can't help feeling that I should be able to take control of it and just be happy! I feel guilty for having this, as I don't want to burden my family with something else – as if there's not already enough stress in my life to deal with. I guess this is where I have to be the strong woman I know I am deep down inside. I know I'm not alone. I know I need to pick up the phone and call someone. I just have to keep telling myself that.

And now my son is awake, and I must dive back into caring for him. I love him dearly. He is the most precious little angel on earth…

Even at that dark, lonely time, I wanted somehow to share what was happening. It began as a personal journal, but as my recovery progressed, it grew into something more. There was a community of women out there who appreciated what I had to say, just as I loved hearing their voices or reading their words. We began to share our stories with each other.

November 2010

The more I talk about Postpartum Depression (PPD), the more I feel better, and the more I realize how common it is. I feel genuinely touched to know how much support I have gotten–from friends and family, and from other mothers alike. It's humbling to know I am not alone in my battle.

Meanwhile, my mommy group had become another big source of light and joy in my life. We appreciated each other and talked frankly, as friends, about the ups and downs of motherhood. In that group, I was a mother of two; most others were on their first child, and many of them felt worried and confused, just as I had felt with Zackery. Sometimes, they would ask me for advice and perspective.

Reclaim the Joy of Motherhood

I will be the first to tell you that I absolutely love giving advice. I don't like bossing people around—I'm not one of those women who bombard fellow mothers with unsolicited instructions on how to correctly care for a baby—but I've come to understand that, by sharing my own experience, I might be able to help another mother improve hers. I love talking to moms and pregnant women about everything having to do with pregnancy and childbirth. I ask a ton of questions, and always try to offer my support. Maybe it comes from my own experience of not being sure what to do with Zackery: When he was an infant, I thought I had to do everything exactly as it was written in the baby books, otherwise I would be a bad mother. But as we struggled to take care of our always-crying son, Will and I started experimenting. We ended up trying everything, and do you know what worked? A little bit of this, a little bit of that. Once we threw strict methods out the door and learned to adapt to the situation at hand, that's when it all started to work.

In my blog circles and in my mommy group, I saw so many new mothers struggling with the ever-widening gap between their expectation of motherhood and the reality they were living. I felt their pain—oh, how deeply I felt that pain. I can't stand to see new moms suffering, and I hate seeing babies suffering because their mother just doesn't know what to do. When that happens, I do have the power to help. I can offer up my experience, and I can offer perspective.

April 2011

I've come to the conclusion that I am definitely a perfectionist. Actually, this is something I've known for quite some time, but today I've decided to own it! I have so many stories I want to share and so many parenting topics I want to write about, but I just can't seem to get started. I am plagued with wanting to write the "perfect" blog post. Well, to that I say... "So long! Here I am! Take it or leave it!" There is no "perfect" when it comes to parenting.

Once I recognized my own perfectionism as a hurdle to overcome, instead of an unattainable standard to live by, I started finding my voice on a more public level. I began openly sharing with moms the things that had worked for me—and I also shared with them the reality Will and I discovered: That parenting is really about being adaptable and flexible. No child is the mirror of a hypothetical in a textbook on mothering. Every moment of every child's life is a discovery, and there is no right or wrong way to deal with that. You just adapt.

When I offered advice to my fellow mothers, it was always with the hope that their life would get a little easier as a result. I love to help. It makes me sleep easier to know that another mother might have been able to find a solution to her problem. But even with that underlying drive and passion for offering advice, I still never thought I had anything particularly special or important to say. It wasn't until people began asking for my opinions and experience that I thought, Hey, maybe I do have something of value to share.

May 2011

I figured it was time to write a little update about how my Postpartum Depression was going. It's been about six months now since I first made the call for help. I've had ups and downs, improvement and decline, but the one constant has been the unwavering support of my family and friends. Without surrounding myself with love and continuing to be open about it, I don't think I would have been able to get through the worst.

I can now say that my anti-depressant medication is stable (and thankfully working). It took several changes in dose, and switching to a different prescription, before I could finally see a light at the end of the dark, dark tunnel. And it was a very gloomy path.

During my most discouraging months, my best friend told me "This isn't you. You aren't a depressed person." She was right! It wasn't me. I am a happy person, and it feels good to finally be headed in that direction again.

I will continue to be open about my journey–both the struggles and the accomplishments. I will continue to stay positive–especially if and when things start to become challenging. I will continue to love and support everyone around me–it's the least I can do for what they have given me. I will continue to be at peace with my internal circumstances–understanding and acknowledging that I did not do this to myself; it is not my fault, I had no control.

Lastly, I will continue to heal myself…

I've mentioned before that, though I haven't read all the books on postpartum disorders, the ones I have read were either dry and clinical, or quite sad. I remember reading Brooke Shields' memoir Down Came The Rain, about her own struggle with PPD. If she can write her story, why can't I? I thought. So, a year or so after my diagnosis, I committed to writing my own book: one written for you, the woman experiencing it. I wanted to offer you hope and joy and a bright future, as well as the tools to reach it. From the bottom of my heart, I hope this book has achieved its goal for at least one woman.

While this book is for you, it helps me heal as well. By writing my story, I validated my experience. My PPD journey is real, not something I made up; it happened, and by writing it down, I accepted that reality on a very deep level and turned it into something positive. This has been one of the most healing choices I have ever made, and one of the most emotionally transformative experiences I have ever had.

Writing about my transformation, my recovery, brought me back at times to where I didn't want to be anymore, and I would find myself crying in the middle of a coffee shop or library. The memories and the pain I had to go through again, to account for every detail I could (or wanted to) remember—it was hard. It was also necessary. I believe that without writing about my experience, I might still be lingering on the threshold of happiness. Now, the most incredible thing has happened: I can delve deeply into those emotions, putting myself right back into the worst of it, so that I can share with an open heart—and then I can snap out of it. By reliving this experience so fully, I am no longer powerless or fearful. I can look the pain in the eye and tell it to disappear.

Writing this book is not the end of my journey. All along, I have been guided by a desire to help and support women. I do not want generation after generation of mothers to go through what I went through, without any idea of how common and treatable

PPD is. I want to drag this syndrome out of the shameful shadows where it has been hiding, and bring it into the light for all to see. I want Postpartum Depression to be talked about as commonly as cancer and diabetes, and I want to see the shame and stigma surrounding it disappear.

January 2012

Life is sometimes hard, and sometimes a billion things come rumbling down the road at us all at the same time. Sometimes all we can do is put on our armor, hunker down, and fight back, knowing it won't last forever. Whatever your circumstances, keep in mind you are NOT them–they do not define you. Try to smile and laugh about it (easier said than done, I know). Take this pledge with me, and I will continue to remind myself, I am not my circumstances–I AM happy!

Ultimately, my biggest inspiration is to work intimately with women. As I began writing this book, I started brainstorming a new endeavor, a program to expand and complement what I've written here by guiding women through the healing journey. I wanted to find a way to offer women advice and perspective, as well as concrete information, recovery strategies, and hope for the future.

At first, I wasn't sure what to call myself in this new role. Yes, I am and will always be an advocate for PPD awareness—but that didn't express the guidance I wanted to offer. Could I be a counselor or a coach? To me, counselors seem to have a higher level of certification and education. Coaches, while they give you encouragement and strategy, haven't necessarily experienced what you are going through. And so, I found the word "mentor"—someone who has been there, done that, and who is willing to share what she has learned.

February 2012

I did something very brave for myself yesterday. I cut my pills in half. HUH? Yes, I am still taking anti-depressant medication. I have wanted to wean myself for several months, but the day I went to the doctor and talked to her about my intention, I literally was in tears because I wasn't ready. How was I ready to be medication-free when I made my appointment, and then be freaked out and terrified to go off them just a few days later? Life is funny that way, and our minds and bodies are extremely intuitive as to what we need. I will say that I have gotten very good at hearing what my body is trying to tell me. I'm not always so good at listening, but my awareness is usually up there, ranking high.

Anyway, as I was saying… I cut my pills in half. Last night.

As the Happy Mommy Mentor, my role is to walk side by side with women through the storms and the darkness, leading you toward the bright horizon where you can reclaim your joy. I promise to be honest and vulnerable, offering you my open heart and everything that I have learned along my own journey. I want to show you that you are not alone, that you have not done anything wrong, and that you will find joy again.

Mentorship and advocacy have given me a new purpose, and it is one that fulfills me on the deepest level. Not only is this process incredibly rewarding as I see mothers reaching new heights and rediscovering their true, happy selves, but the practice of mentoring you also helps keep me on the right track. I know that I will never again descend to that level of depression because of the tools I have put in place for myself. But in order to stay happy, I need to practice what I preach, consistently. When I teach these methods, I also keep myself accountable. My healing is an ongoing process that will never truly end, and the more I work with other women, the more I continue working on myself. I know the more I write, the more I talk about it, the more I share from my heart, the easier it will be for me to stay on this path. It is something I will undoubtedly have to work at for years to come. Thankfully, I have the awareness now of what I need to do to self-sustain and never retreat back into depression.

I find myself more aware of my moods, my cycle, and the triggers that affect me negatively. I have a newfound connection to my deeper, spiritual self. I have built upon the strength and courage within me, constantly working towards my ultimate goal of helping others. I continue to write, talk, and share openly, from my heart, about my experience with Postpartum Depression, and I am no longer hesitant or ashamed to mention it. The more I share, the more I heal, and I will never give that up.

August 2012

It's been a while since I've written about PPD–Postpartum Depression, that is. I had it, I had it bad, but I got through it. It's over and done. I'm better, and now I just get to deal with normal everyday stresses (not sure which is better–having an excuse or not). Possible excuses aside, I wanted to write about my PPD. I've written about it before, but it's been a while, so here goes again.

I'm officially 100% off my meds. I can ignore the "current medications" box on forms at the doctor's office. I can forget about having to remember to take my happy pill. It feels good to not be putting anything unnecessary into my body (I do enough of that with the wine and food I indulge in). I feel stronger, more like the woman I know I am. I'm gaining my confidence back, feeling more empowered and ready to get back into the "real" world.

Community. It's all about community and relationships. Everything is: family, friends, your health, even the relationship you have with yourself. Knowing you don't "feel" right is a big awareness towards the relationship you have with your body, mind, and spirit. When I was in the depths of my PPD, I knew I wasn't myself. I just didn't know how to get myself back because it had been so long since I knew who I was that I had forgotten who my normal self was. I know who I am now, and who I am has changed. I've shifted, but in a good way. Flexibility is more than a physical measurement, and especially as a mother (you all know what I'm talking about), we have to be flexible. When your child has a fever in the middle of the night and you're supposed to watch someone else's child the next morning, you both have to be flexible. Plans change. Things happen. Life goes on.

I'm happy to be on the path I'm on now. I'm excited about my next step. Baby steps, but a step forward nonetheless. I'm excited to have the opportunity to help others going through PPD. I'm glad that my horrible, deep, dark abyss had meaning. And what I'm most happy about is being happy again!

One of my (many) next steps, a vision, is to help facilitate better screening from the doctors for Postpartum Depression. Not just the OB's, but the pediatricians and family doctors as well – the doctors who actually see new mothers at the time when they might be experiencing PPD.

I don't mean to pass judgment on the way the system works now, other than that it just doesn't work. When a woman doesn't see her OB after six weeks postpartum, how is he/she supposed to properly screen for PPD?

If we trained all doctors better on the symptoms and signs of PPD, and on how to properly screen those women who raise a red flag at an office visit for their child, I believe the number of women diagnosed with PPD might actually increase. But that would not necessarily be a bad thing: It would mean we could start helping mothers heal that much faster. Less lengthy suffering, less stigma, less shame and guilt that a woman has to carry.

Having women feel comfortable speaking out and getting help for this common affliction: that would really make me happy. I hope that, over the years ahead, we continue to see things moving in this direction. I will do everything I can to support a positive change.

CHAPTER SEVENTEEN

Happy Mommy Mentor

"I don't think you ever stop giving. I really don't. I think it's an ongoing process. And it's not just about being able to write a check. It's being able to touch somebody's life."

- Oprah Winfrey

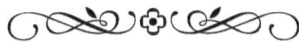

Now that you have made your way to the end of this book, I hope you will give me the opportunity to work with you as you continue healing and building the new life you always wanted. I'd like to tell you more about my program for women going through Postpartum Depression: The HAPPY Mommy Method™.

It's a five-step process to help you find happiness, confidence and joy in motherhood. I'm offering several different ways to work through that process, but the basic experience is the same: I will personally guide you through each of these steps.

HOPE: *Finding your hope for happiness, and your vision of what life will be like after Postpartum Depression.*

ACTION: *Making changes and taking steps toward your vision.*

PROCESS: *Creating the habits and structure that help you heal faster and more completely, for a lifetime of continued happiness.*

PHYSICAL: *Focusing on physical wellbeing so your body can support your healing process.*

YOU: *Learning to put yourself first, so you can be at your best for others.*

I am so incredibly excited to share this process with you. It's deeply important to me. When I was healing from my own Postpartum Depression, I was lucky enough to have an amazing support network—Will, my friends, my doula—but I never had that one person: the woman who had been through it. As supportive as all those people have been to me—and I would never trade them for a second—they can never understand exactly what it was like, because they simply have never felt it. One of the major reasons I created The HAPPY Mommy Method™ was so I can be that person to you, and women like you. You might have a wonderful support network like I did, or you might be feeling all alone in the world—but you have me, and I will be here to guide you.

When I think about the possibility of stopping my work as The HAPPY Mommy Mentor, I feel a little empty inside. To stop would be to let myself and other moms down. I truly feel that this is my calling, more than architecture ever was. It is what I am meant to be doing right now, and I am driven to do it. The number one thing that gets me out of bed every morning with a smile is the thought of spending time with my boys. But when I have the house to myself and a free day to work on my programs, I'm always excited. I love working on updates and tweaks to make things go more smoothly, creating new modules and exercises, and designing different ways to help the women who have placed their trust in me.

I refuse to believe that women going through PPD need to suffer alone. I won't let it happen, at least not where I have the power to make a difference. I want to help strip away the layers of stigma and remorse that surround women who have done nothing wrong. I live to empower mothers to bravely reclaim their true selves and their joy.

There's another important thing for you to know: I live by this method. It is a practice that I devised through my own research and development, and it worked for me—and continues to work for me, because I continue to follow it. In fact, if I ever get busy or distracted and don't stick with my program, I notice the effects. I can sense myself getting in a slump and becoming cranky, and I can see how it affects the people around me. And so, this program is a lifestyle for me. I live by it, and it keeps me buoyant, bright, and joyful. I know that, following this program, I will never lose myself in depression again.

How Does The HAPPY Mommy Method Work?

My programs are constantly changing and evolving organically, and each person's details will differ depending on their circumstance. I guarantee that each of my programs will be specifically designed to help you transform your life with the five steps I have outlined. And with each of the programs, it will be a give-and-take process: In order for it to work, you will need to open your heart and do the work to create healing in your life.

Many women will find their transformation through a teleseminar program—a regular phone call with me during which we will explore each of the five steps as a group, and you will complete homework assignments on your own time that will help you find your unique solutions and tools for growth.

Some women will choose to work with me one-on-one in an extended mentorship program: a series of private phone calls where you can bare your soul to me in a safe place, and I will guide you along the path of recovery.

In other cases, I might see you at an event, either as the leader or as a speaker. I also host retreats and VIP programs. If you are interested in finding out more, I hope you will get in touch to find out what programs might work best for your situation.

Every single program will go through the same process, and every program will have similar homework assignments. While the healing process and the commitment to yourself will be the same for every woman, each program will differ in the level of intimacy, personal time, and access you have with me. I can't emphasize enough that the homework and self-care is your responsibility, and it is the most important part of your recovery. I can only give you my own experience, knowledge, and encouragement from the bottom of my heart—your progress along the path will be up to you.

However, I promise to you that everything I know, everything I can share, every way I can help you is yours for the taking. My heart is open to every woman going through Postpartum Depression, and I will do everything I can to give you the guidance you need.

Who Is This Method For?

I designed my programs for all new mothers—not necessarily first-time mothers, but mothers with young children—who seek joy and healing. If you have been diagnosed with PPD, or feel you might have it, I believe you need to consider this program. I hope you will at least reach out, so we can talk. It might mean the difference between a life of joy and a life of emotional struggle.

However, I also understand that some of you reading this book are not directly suffering from PPD, but are suffering because someone close to you is in need of help. If one of your friends or loved ones is going through PPD or seems to be going through it, I can offer you my research and recommendations for ways to help them.

I cannot solve depression. I am simply giving you the tools to work through the healing process using self-care and natural methods. My programs are intended to accompany the treatment your doctor recommends—whatever that is. I hope that some doctors will recommend my program as well, or even as an alternative to treatment in certain cases. Ultimately, it is up to you and your doctor, and The HAPPY Mommy Method™ is just one facet of recovery.

When you are considering whether this method is for you, don't just think about the challenges or difficulties of going through it—think about the danger and cost of not doing it. Do you want to stay sad, possibly endangering your health and your baby's? Of course not. I will not try to scare you with the dangers of not getting help, but there are serious risks, and you have the power to avoid them. The choice is yours.

How Can I Prepare For This Program?

There is absolutely nothing you need to do to prepare, except to commit. Commit to having an open heart, to being vulnerable, and to doing the work. You can visit my website or send me an email right now. The hardest step is the first one, and I appreciate what it takes to make that first step.

If you are preparing to enter one of my programs, the one additional positive action you might want to take is to schedule your "me time"—something I have talked about several times in this book—to focus on your recovery, to have a protected space for your sessions, and to create a quiet environment so you can do your homework. You will need to create a space and time with no interruptions and no kids—don't laugh! Just find the quietest environment available, so you can truly focus on yourself.

If that is not possible yet, don't let it stop you from getting in touch. Every problem can be overcome, and I hope I can help you with this one. In the long run, though, every single person in the world needs time to be on their own, and new parents need it most of all. Finding a way to make this happen for yourself will make a big difference in your mental clarity, no matter what.

The greatest value of this project, for me, will always be the way it has transformed my life. I am so grateful and blessed to have found a path out of the darkness; now I know that all I have to do is keep putting one foot in front of the other. Life may never be easy, but from now on, I know it will be happy.

CONCLUSION

Joy – Just The Other Side Of PPD

"You must learn to be still in the midst of activity and to be vibrantly alive in repose."

- *Indira Gandhi*

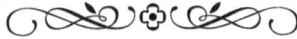

You're a big girl, Pamela, I tell myself firmly. Don't cry. You don't need to do that any more. Get it together, you'll be fine. But as the line in front of me gets shorter and shorter, my anxiety and fear build to a frantic, pulsing drumbeat in my chest.

Stop it! I tell myself, but it is no use. The woman in front of me steps away, and it is just me now, facing my fear. Giant, hot tears burst from my eyes. I put my head in my hands. The people on either side of me take my arms, gently, for support.

"Just breathe," somebody says. Just breathe, I say to myself. I take a deep breath and step forward bravely with my bare foot.

Onto a field of sharp, broken glass.

Reclaim the Joy of Motherhood

I am at a retreat in Tucson, Arizona, and today we are challenging ourselves on the very deepest level. Would you walk on glass? Today, I have watched a hundred women do just that. This doesn't make it easy, not even a little. But everyone else seems to be holding it together, even having fun. Why am I crying?

Four slow, calculated steps later, my foot makes contact with the velvety soft grass, whose blades cushion my toes like the softest pillow I can imagine. I smile from ear to ear. And then I burst into tears all over again.

My name is Pamela Zimmer, and I'm a crier. But you know what? That's just who I am. It doesn't make me any less strong, intelligent, or brave. I can walk over glass with tears in my eyes! Can you?

Recently, a friend helped me uncover the psychological conflict that seems to contribute to my outbursts of tears. It's a battle being fought in my head: I want to do something incredible and life-altering, but a little voice says, *Are you crazy? You can't do that!*

Luckily, I happen to have another little voice in my head. *Oh yeah?* it says. *Just watch me!*

You can't start your own architecture firm!

Oh yeah? Watch me.

You're not really going to get married, are you?

Just watch me.

You'll never be able to go through childbirth naturally, with no drugs.

Oh yeah? Watch me.

You can't turn your Postpartum Depression struggle into a book and a program!

WATCH ME.

The bottom line is, I can do anything I want. You can, too. There will always be fear; there will often be a field of broken glass to walk over. But when that little voice in your head tells you that you can't do it, just prove it wrong. Take the first step, even with tears in your eyes.

Growing up, and even as an adult, my existence was governed by an ideal of perfection. Like an invisible puppeteer, my looming perfectionism pulled my strings and dictated so many of the actions I took. I always thought that was a good thing: I am a driven person, always eager to achieve as much as I can in life, and it always seemed to me that, if I tried hard enough, I might embody that image of perfection. But ultimately, it was my perfectionism that made me inflexible, unable to adapt to the changes in my life. I was bound by those strings, and the only way to survive was to cut them and figure out how to live my way.

In the process of recovering from Postpartum Depression, I learned so much. I learned that it's okay to ask for help—that asking for help doesn't make you weak, it makes you strong. I learned to love and accept my strengths, my weaknesses, and my triggers. I learned to share those things with the people who love me, so they can look out for me and help me correct my course before I wander off a cliff.

Most importantly, I learned that I can't be in control of everything—that the more I try to be in control, the crazier and more stressed I will get. Instead of controlling the external things that happen to me, I have learned to control my reactions to those things. After all, you can't really do anything about what happens to you, but you can decide what to do about it.

If you come over to my house, it might be a little messy. I've learned to let go of some of the little things that used to drive me crazy because there are other things that are simply more important. Do I get irritated when there are water spots on the counter and graham cracker crumbs on the floor? Of course. Does it kill me? No. Are my kids happy? Have they eaten? Yes and yes! We will get to the crumbs.

My home truly is a happy one, and I don't say that to brag—I say it because it is something I know that you can have, too. When people come over, they notice it. When I get up in the morning and walk into the kitchen to see my boys, their faces light up. They are so good. Yes, they drive me crazy at times, and yes, I have to discipline them. But I am a good mom, and I'm confident in my decisions, and those boys will grow up to be good men.

Will has never let me down, and though we are no longer starry-eyed newlyweds, we support each other from our souls. We still have rebuilding to do, but we have learned to share our dreams and passions with each other, and we are each genuinely excited for the other's ambitions and achievements.

I think about my mother every day. It doesn't scare or hurt me anymore. I talk to my mom all the time, and I know she is listening. She may never get to hold and be with her grandsons, but she is calm and at peace. She knows we are happy. And when I talk to her about all the things I have accomplished and all the shining dreams that lie ahead, I know she is beaming. Somewhere very close by, my mother is proud of me.

I love being ambitious. That is one part of me that will never, ever change. I will always be driven to do great things and change the world. It is something I truly love about myself. After all this time, all these struggles and victories, I have finally learned the most important thing: I don't need to be perfect and do it all, but I don't need to sit idly by and watch the world turn, either. I can do amazing things, and now I can do them more completely and successfully, because now I honor myself and take care of myself first. It is okay to be afraid, okay to make mistakes, okay to cry. In the end, those things have no effect on my life. They are little things, and I have learned to let them go.

Dear reader, whoever you are, I want to thank you for going on this journey with me. I hope that, through the course of this book, you have found new hope and even some joy, and a reason to believe that life can and will get better. I am excited for the things you will achieve in the months and years ahead, when you cut the bonds that hold you back, and begin to act as your true and unique self. I believe in your strength, as I believe in your power to overcome anything in life.

I have worked hard to give you knowledge, tools, and perspective that you can use to recreate your world. From here, only you know what shape your creation will take. I believe it will be beautiful, shining with light as you hang new stars in the heavens. But right now, if your sky is still dark, remember that you are not alone. Reach out your hand, and I will be there. We can face this together, and soon the heavens will be dotted with pinpoints of light, all shining for you.

Dear reader, I know from the very bottom of my heart that your future is bright. And from the bottom of my heart, I hope I have helped you to glimpse it.

APPENDIX

Resource Guide

"Let us tenderly and kindly cherish, therefore, the means of knowledge. Let us dare to read, think, speak, and write."

- John Adams

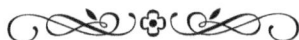

The information in these pages is not the final word on any of these topics. I am not a medical doctor, a scientist, or licensed counselor, but I do consider myself an expert and I have done my homework. This chapter represents all the information I found useful as I struggled to understand my Postpartum Depression. I hope it will help you on your own journey of discovery and learning.

All of these links and more are also available on my website: www.PamelaZimmer.com.

How To Reach Me

I am here for you, and I hope you will reach out. I am happy to speak with you individually on the phone or via email, and I would also love to have you join my mentoring program, The HAPPY Mommy Method™. This is a program designed for women like you, who are ready to begin a journey of healing.

Reclaim the Joy of Motherhood

On your journey, as your mentor I will guide you through
the five steps to help you find confidence, happiness and joy
in motherhood. However, you do not need to sign up for the
program, and I won't pressure you to do so. I am here to support
you, no matter what.

Please get in touch with me at: info@pamelazimmer.com

Getting Help Right Now

If you need help now, please call a hotline number. No matter what
you are feeling, someone will be there to listen.

- The Postpartum Support International Warmline:
  1-800-944-4PPD (800 944 4773)

- The National Suicide Prevention Lifeline:
  1-800-273-TALK (800 273 8255)

- The Childhelp National Child Abuse Hotline:
  1-800-4-A-CHILD (800 422 4453)

You can also fill in the blanks here with some numbers to call when
things are very hard:

My doctor: _____

My counselor/mentor/therapist: _____

Friend(s) to call: _____

Finding Community

You are not alone! Millions of other women know what you are feeling. When you feel like nobody understands what is happening to you, you can reach out and find those women, waiting to help and support you. Here are some good places to start.

- Online PPD Support Group
  PPDsupportpage.com

- PPD Support Groups in the U.S. and Canada
  PostpartumProgress.com
  Postpartum Progress maintains a list of support groups for mothers.

- Postpartum Support International
  Postpartum.net
  Find PPD groups and sources of help in your area.

- National Association of Mothers' Centers
  MothersCenter.org
  Find centers dedicated to caring for mothers.

If you are having trouble finding a group in your area, try calling your local church or community center. Many times, there will be support groups available that are not advertised online. You can also talk to a counselor or to your doctor about finding local groups.

Information You Can Trust

When you're looking for information on the Internet, it can be hard to know which sources to trust. Beware of websites with exaggerated statistics or dramatic stories. Look for websites created by medical organizations, non-profits, and qualified experts. Here are some of the websites and resources I found to be helpful, legitimate, and well-researched.

- Postpartum Support International (Postpartum.net)

- PostpartumProgress.org

- BabyCenter.com

- WebMD.com

- MayoClinic.com

- PubMed Health (NCBI.NLM.NIH.GOV/PubMedHealth)

- MedicineNet.com

- WomensHealth.gov

- PostpartumMen.com

Collected Research

The following are summaries of the information I uncovered through my own research and discovery. I urge you to follow up by doing your own searching, as well as by talking to your doctor. This information should help you get started.

What is Postpartum Depression?

According to the National Library of Medicine, Postpartum Depression is defined as "moderate to severe depression in a woman after she has given birth. It may occur soon after delivery or up to a year later. Most of the time, it occurs within the first 3 months after delivery."[12] Postpartum Depression is a temporary medical condition which, if left untreated, can last up to a year or more, having significant negative effects on the relationship of the entire family. It is not a sign of weakness, it is not anything that can be fully predicted and/or prevented, and it is not anyone's fault.

Postpartum Depression does not discriminate. It can happen to any woman, regardless of age, race, culture, social status, or income level. It can also occur in women who have already had children, in women who have adopted, and even after miscarriage or stillbirth. Surprisingly, it can also occur in men, affecting up to 10 percent of new fathers.[13]

Statistically, up to 80 percent of new mothers experience some kind of mood-related symptoms during the first two weeks following childbirth.[14] This is typically called the Baby Blues, and it usually goes away on its own within the first two to three weeks. When these symptoms persist, worsen, or become more severe and/or frequent, this is called Postpartum Depression (PPD).

Postpartum Depression does not always start immediately after birth. The symptoms of PPD can begin several weeks after childbirth, after what would be the normal Baby Blues period, and can even begin months later. Typically, onset is within the first year. There are no laboratory tests to diagnose Postpartum Depression, though it is the most common complication associated with childbirth.

When I was first researching Postpartum Depression just before my own diagnosis, I found many statistics stating that one in eight women suffer from Postpartum Depression. Years later, I have found sources saying that statistic has increased to one in seven women[15] , and even up to 20 percent (1 in 5). Some researchers believe (and I tend to agree with them) that the percentage has risen because awareness of PPD is increasing, and women that previously would not have reported it are beginning to speak up. Women are afraid to talk about Postpartum Depression, even to their doctors. Instead, they remain silent, suffering alone without help. I strive to help change that.

There is no single cause for Postpartum Depression. Hormone changes alone are not always triggers of PPD in new mothers. External circumstances can also play a role: varying factors associated with lifestyle, environment (both at home and at work), financial situation, family relationships, and any recent experience of trauma or grief. Sometimes, Postpartum Depression is merely a complication of giving birth.

PPD Symptoms

A mother with Postpartum Depression may find it hard to function well, or to adequately care for and bond with her baby. Some women also believe that they may harm themselves or their baby, which is why it is so important to talk to your doctor or care provider about your symptoms. The symptoms of Postpartum Depression mirror those of any other kind of depression that may occur at other times in life. Those symptoms may include, but are not limited to, the following:

- Feelings of hopelessness, or helplessness
- Feelings of worry or anxiety
- Feelings of sadness or crying all the time
- Feelings of guilt or shame
- Irritability or mood swings
- Lack of focus or difficulty concentrating
- Fatigue or exhaustion
- Trouble sleeping
- Changes in appetite
- Lack of interest in activities you would normally enjoy
- Feeling withdrawn or disconnected
- Headaches, backaches, or other body aches
- Problems doing everyday tasks at home or work

- Inability or lack of desire to care for your baby or yourself

- Negative feelings towards your baby

- Fear of being alone with your baby

- Thoughts of harming your baby, your other children, and/or yourself

- Thoughts of death or suicide

Even if you aren't experiencing any of these symptoms, if you feel like something is wrong, or if you just don't feel like yourself, the best thing you can do is to talk to your doctor or care provider. It might not be anything, or it might be some form of Postpartum Depression, Postpartum Anxiety, or even Postpartum Psychosis. All of these illnesses are real, some more common than others, and with expert help can all be treated.

It does not hurt to be open about any changes you notice. The worst that can happen is that you might get help for something early on, before it becomes serious. The sooner you get help, the sooner you will begin to feel better.

Risk Factors

Although there is no way to definitively predict or prevent Postpartum Depression, some women may be more likely to get it than others. One of the strongest predictors that a woman might get Postpartum Depression is depression or anxiety during pregnancy, especially in the third trimester.[16] Other risk factors include, but are not limited to:

- Prior or family history of depression or anxiety

- Difficulties with a spouse or partner

- Stressful life events such as losing a job, moving, or the death or illness of a loved one

- Financial distress

- Lack of social support or adequate help with childcare

- Caring for a child with behavioral or temperamental challenges

- Low self-esteem

- Age (under age twenty)

- Marital status (single people are more susceptible)

- Unplanned or unwanted pregnancy

- Difficult or traumatic birth experience

- Alcohol, drug or tobacco abuse

- Having a sick or colicky baby

These risk factors do not automatically cause Postpartum Depression. Some women never experience Postpartum Depression, despite having many of the above factors present in their daily lives. Other women might get Postpartum Depression with only one risk factor, or sometimes even none, present. It is important to remember that each woman is different.

Research also shows that, if a mother has experienced PPD with one child, she has about a sevemty-five percent chance of experiencing it again. "It seems to be a 'crapshoot,'" says wellness consultant Stacey Glaesmann. "A mother of five could have had PPD with the first child and then not get it again, could have it with all five, or could have it with only some of her children. It depends on her life situation at the time."

Glaesmann conducted a study to unearth potential risk factors for developing PPD, and her results showed that the most telling factor was what the mother thought of her baby's temperament. "If the mother perceived her child to have a 'difficult' temperament, she was more likely to develop a PPMD." However, this does not mean that the mother of an "easy" baby isn't also at risk for PPD.

There is never a need to feel ashamed, guilty, or embarrassed about being diagnosed with or having Postpartum Depression. It is no different than needing medical attention for an infection or other illness. Though it is not often openly talked about (unfortunately, sometimes not even between medical professionals), it is real.

Screening Tools

Although there is no single test to diagnose Postpartum Depression, one of the most common tools used to screen for Postpartum Depression is the Edinburgh Postnatal Depression Scale (EPDS). It is a series of ten questions that a new mother can answer based on how she has been feeling within the past seven days. Her responses may help determine if she is at risk for Postpartum Depression, and consequently may warrant further examination and inquiry.

You can find a copy of the test in Chapter Five, "What is Happening to You?". You can also find the test and further information on my website, www.PamelaZimmer.com.

Medications

NOTE: This section is not intended to take the place of professional or medical advice. Medication is not always right for everyone. Always talk to your doctor or care provider before starting or stopping any drug, whether over-the-counter or prescription.

Studies have shown that the most common antidepressant medications prescribed to breastfeeding women with Postpartum Depression are selective-serotonin reuptake inhibitors (or SSRIs), specifically Zoloft (Sertraline) and Paxil (Paroxetine). These medications are considered safe for nursing infants. Both of these drugs have levels within or under what is considered safe for breastfeeding, and in many cases they were completely undetectable.

"If a risk/benefit analysis shows that the mother would benefit more from taking an SSRI than the potential risk to her baby, then I will recommend she see a medical doctor," Glaesmann says. Multiple studies argue that the baby is less at risk from the insignificant levels of these chemicals in a mother's breast milk than if the mother remains untreated for depression.

Each mother is unique: while some may have a stronger desire to continue to breastfeed while taking antidepressant medication, others may choose to cease nursing. There is no right or wrong.

Each mother should be given equal respect and support of her decision.

If a mother is not breastfeeding her infant, for whatever reason, either through choice or circumstance, the options for antidepressant medication increase. Your doctor or care provider can discuss these options with you.

All medications and drugs, both over-the-counter and prescription, can present side effects. Not everyone experiences or reacts to a medication in the same way, which is why it is vitally important to tell your doctor or care provider about any side effects you may be experiencing. The benefits of taking anti-depressant medications usually outweigh any negative side effects; however, there are instances when you may choose to try a different medication. In some cases, the positive effects of an antidepressant medication might decline over time, in which case you should discuss the possibility of increasing your dosage or switching to a new medication.

Breathing Meditation

This is the breathing meditation I have developed and that I referred to back in Chapter Nine. It works! Use this whenever you need to. I have also made a recording of this meditation, which you can download at PamelaZimmer.com.

Find a comfortable, quiet spot, either inside or outside, where you can be fully present and free to relax, without distractions or interruptions.

Begin by positioning yourself so your feet are flat and touching the surface beneath you, allowing the energy of the earth to ground you.

Close your eyes softly and focus your attention on your body, your chest, as it moves up and down, in and out with each breath. Begin to slow your breath, making each inhale longer than the last, and each exhale full and complete, releasing all tension from your body and all thoughts from your mind.

Continue the focus on your breath until it is steady and slow, breathing in and out, inhaling and exhaling, calmly and completely, flowing and full. Keep this pattern of breathing throughout this exercise. If you find your mind wandering, come back to your breath until you are once again focused on breathing steady and slow, calmly and completely, flowing and full. You may come back to this as often as you need or want to.

Bring your awareness to the soles of your feet. Feel how the earth is holding them. With each inhale, feel the energy of the earth as it freely flows through the bottoms of your feet up into and throughout your entire body. Notice your toes. Notice how relaxed they are. Feel the tension drain from your toes, through the bottoms of your feet. With each exhale, let the earth take all tension away.

Move your awareness now to your legs. Your calves and your shins, your knees, your thighs. Notice how relaxed your legs are, how loose your muscles are. With each inhale, feel the energy of the earth flow up through the bottoms of your feet, up your shins, past your knees and into your thighs. With each exhale, let all your tension go. Feel the tension drain down your legs, through the bottoms of your feet, into the earth.

Now shift your awareness to your hips and pelvis, your lower abdomen. Notice how relaxed they are, how open and free. With each inhale, feel the energy of the earth flow up through the bottoms of your feet, up your legs and into your abdomen. With each exhale, let all of your tension go. Feel the tightness drain down your legs, through the bottoms of your feet, into the earth.

Bring your awareness up now to your torso, your stomach, your chest, your back. Notice your ribcage and spine. Notice how aligned and relaxed they are. With each inhale, feel the energy of the earth flow up through the bottoms of your feet, up your legs, through your abdomen, up your back and chest and up to the top of your spine. With each exhale, release all tension. Feel the tension drain down each vertebrae, down your pelvis, into your legs and out the bottoms of your feet, into the earth.

Move your awareness up your body to your neck and shoulders and into your arms and fingers. Notice how relaxed they are. Feel how loose they are. With each inhale, feel the energy of the earth flow up through the bottoms of your feet, up your legs, through your pelvis and torso, up your spine and into your neck and shoulders. Let the tension go. Feel your shoulders drop and your fingers relax. With each exhale, feel the tension drain down your neck into your spine, into your abdomen, down your legs and through the bottoms of your feet, into the earth.

Turn your awareness now to your face. Notice your jaw, your

ears, your lips, your cheeks, your forehead. Feel how relaxed they are. With each inhale, feel the energy of the earth flow up through the bottoms of your feet, up your legs, your abdomen, your torso, your neck and into your face, all the way up to the crown of your head. Let the tension go. Feel your face soften. With each exhale, feel the tension drain, out of your face and head, down your neck and spine, all the way down your body into your legs and the bottoms of your feet, into the earth.

Focus your awareness now on your entire body. Notice any areas where there might still be tension. With your inhale, bring the energy up into that area, and then exhale to release the tension. Feel it drain out through the bottoms of your feet, into the earth.

You are now fully relaxed. Enjoy this full relaxation for a moment. Be present. Just breathe, steady and slow, calmly and completely, flowing and full.

When you are ready, gradually bring your awareness back to your surroundings, back to your body position, and gently open your eyes.

REFERENCES

1 http://www.nlm.nih.gov/medlineplus/postpartumdepression.html

2 http://www.webmd.com/depression/physical-symptoms

3 http://www.postpartumprogress.com/the-symptoms-of-postpartum-depression-anxiety-in-plain-mama-english

4 I am not a medical professional, and am not qualified to give medical advice of any kind. This represents my own research, and I believe it can help you, but you should always talk to your own doctor or care provider about your unique situation and symptoms.

5 Cox, J.L., Holden, J.M., and Sagovsky, R. 1987. Detection of postnatal depression: Development of the 10-item Edinburgh Postnatal Depression Scale. British Journal of Psychiatry 150:782-786.

6 K. L. Wisner, B. L. Parry, C. M. Piontek, Postpartum Depression N Engl J Med vol. 347, No 3, July 18, 2002, 194-199.

7 http://www.ncbi.nlm.nih.gov/pubmedhealth/PMH0004481/

8 http://www.apa.org/pi/women/resources/reports/postpartum-dep.aspx

9 http://www.postpartummen.com/

10 http://americanpregnancy.org/firstyearoflife/babyblues.htm

11 http://www.babycenter.com/0_postpartum-depression-and-anxiety_227.bc

12 http://www.ncbi.nlm.nih.gov/pubmedhealth/PMH0004481/

13 http://www.postpartummen.com/

14 http://americanpregnancy.org/firstyearoflife/babyblues.htm

15 http://www.apa.org/pi/women/resources/reports/postpartum-dep.aspx

16 http://www.babycenter.com/0_postpartum-depression-and-anxiety_227.bc